# Australia's Toxic Medical Culture

Vicki Adele Pascoe

# Australia's Toxic Medical Culture

International Medical Graduates
and Structural Power

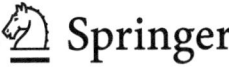 Springer

Vicki Adele Pascoe
Principal Researcher
Independent Education Consultancy
Adelaide, SA, Australia

ISBN 978-981-13-2425-3        ISBN 978-981-13-2426-0   (eBook)
https://doi.org/10.1007/978-981-13-2426-0

Library of Congress Control Number: 2018953305

This Springer imprint is published by the registered company Springer Nature Singapore Pte Ltd.
The registered company address is: 152 Beach Road, #21-01/04 Gateway East, Singapore 189721, Singapore

*This book is dedicated to the memory of Professor Steve Redhead: Ultimate Scholar, Consummate Professional and Perfect Gentleman, sadly missed, RIP.*

# Acknowledgements

I wish to thank the many voices who contributed to this study, for gifting your time and sharing lived experiences. Without you, this story could not be told, and this book would not exist.

# Contents

# Acronyms

| | |
|---|---|
| ABS | Australian Bureau of Statistics |
| ACCC | Australian Competition and Consumer Commission |
| ACRRM | Australian College of Rural and Remote Medicine |
| ADTOA | Australian Doctors Trained Overseas Association |
| AHPRA | Australian Health Practitioner Regulation Agency |
| AHWOC | Australian Health Workforce Officials Committee |
| AIDA | Australian Indigenous Doctors' Association |
| AIHW | Australian Institute of Health and Welfare |
| AMA | Australian Medical Association |
| AMC | Australian Medical Council |
| AMSA | Australian Medical Students' Association |
| ANZAC | Australia and New Zealand Army Corps |
| AOA | Australian Orthopaedic Association |
| AON | Area of Need |
| APS | Australian Public Service |
| ARRWAG | Australian Rural & Remote Workforce Agencies Group |
| BMA | British Medical Association |
| CAM | Complementary and Alternative Medicine |
| COAG | Council of Australian Governments |
| DWS | District of Workforce Shortage |
| ECFMG | Educational Commission for Foreign Medical Graduates |
| ELP | English Language Proficiency |
| EPIC | Electronic Portfolio of International Credentials |
| EU | European Union |
| FACRRM | Fellow Australian College of Rural and Remote Medicine |
| FGP | Focus Group Participant |
| FRACGP | Fellow Royal Australian College of General Practitioners |
| GP | General Practitioner |
| HCCA | Health Care Consumers' Association |
| HPARA | Health Practitioners Australia Reform Association |

| IELTS | International English Language Testing System |
|-------|----------------------------------------------|
| IMG | International Medical Graduate |
| IRO | International Refugee Organisation |
| MBA | Medical Board of Australia |
| MP | Member of Parliament |
| NRHA | National Rural Health Alliance |
| OSTAN | Overseas Trained Specialist Anaesthetists Network |
| OTD | Overseas Trained Doctor |
| PESCI | Pre-Employment Structured Clinical Interview |
| RACGP | Royal Australian College of General Practitioners |
| RACS | Royal Australasian College of Surgeons |
| RHWA | Rural Health Workforce Agency |
| SCU | Special Category Visa |
| SIM | Subscriber Information Module |
| UBC | University of British Colombia |
| UKIP | UK Independence Party |
| WDOMS | World Directory of Medical Schools |
| WHO | World Health Organisation |
| WPR | What's the Problem Represented to be Approach |

# List of Tables

# Introduction: Welcome to Australia, the Land of a Fair Go for All

> Australia is the 'lucky country' which still resonates in the minds and the actions of many people here and worldwide. 'Australia' is the land beyond the border (the place that exploited peoples try to reach, and older Australians are nostalgic about)… Australia continues to be perceived from outside as a relatively safe haven. (Tulloch and Lupton 2003, p. 41)
>
> We have to stamp out medical racism before it takes hold. Overseas trained doctors do not practice inferior medicine. Nor are they less committed to patient care. (Haikerwal 2005, p. 5)

In 2003, Dr Jayant Patel moved to Bundaberg Queensland to take up an appointment as Director of Surgery at the Bundaberg Base Hospital. The initial conception for this book was triggered by what became the Dr Patel tragedy. Reported by a whistle-blower nurse, it was alleged that between 2003 and 2005, 30 patients died while under his care. Dr Patel was accused of negligence and was eventually convicted of manslaughter, grievous bodily harm and fraud (Keim et al. 2013). As a result, Dr Patel attracted the nickname 'Dr Death'. Dr Patel, an International Medical Graduate, was born in Jamnagar India where he studied medicine. Dr Patel subsequently undertook further surgical training in the USA and became a US citizen.

The ramifications from the Bundaberg tragedy were widespread, not only were there families in Bundaberg who suffered loss of life or loss of quality of life due to medical mistakes, but it seemed that medical doctors across Australia, particularly those trained overseas and of Indian appearance, were being subjected to abuse (Haikerwal 2005). Hostility towards IMGs surfaced from within the Australian community generally and there was a growing perception that IMG qualifications and skills were substandard.

Remembering this case, I was disturbed by a speech made to the National Press Club in Canberra in July 2005. In his speech, the then president of the Australian Medical Association (AMA) Dr Murkesh Haikerwal (an IMG himself) made the observation that Australia, as a result of the Dr Patel case, was experiencing, 'medical racism'. Dr Haikerwal (2005) stated:

> Because of the Patel case, doctors with funny names, accents, coloured skin and different backgrounds are getting a hard time. Some patients are avoiding them, some patients are

© Springer Nature Singapore Pte Ltd. 2019
V. A. Pascoe, *Australia's Toxic Medical Culture*,
https://doi.org/10.1007/978-981-13-2426-0_1

abusing them…we cannot allow honest, highly skilled doctors to be made pariahs in the communities they are committed to serving…because of the negligence of others, they are bearing a burden that isn't theirs. They are under scrutiny for getting a medical degree from overseas, or for having darker skin, or a different faith, or English as a second language. (Haikerwal 2005, p. 3)

I became interested in what IMGs could be experiencing as a result of the Patel case. This interest only further enticed me to want to explore how IMGs experience living and working in Australian communities generally. One of the first things I noticed was the seeming interchangeable use of the terms overseas trained doctors (OTD) and International Medical Graduates (IMGs). Throughout this book, I will refer to participants and others as IMGs, except when quoting from literature which sometimes refers to these doctors as overseas trained doctors (OTDs) (notably the terms of reference for the 2012 Parliamentary Inquiry). I have followed the preferred terminology recommended by the Australian Medical Council (AMC) below:

> Over the years considerable confusion has arisen regarding the classification of overseas trained doctors because of the different terminology used. The most common term - Overseas Trained Doctors (OTDs) was considered in the mid-1990's to imply some value judgement and was gradually replaced by the term International Medical Graduates (IMGs). This classification is now the international standard terminology…. (Australian Medical Council (AMC) 2012, Submission 42 p. 4)

Before I could appreciate the experiences of IMGs, I needed to know much more about the practice of medicine and the role of a medical practitioner in Australia. The structure and operation of the Australian health system was my base starting point.

## The Australian Health System

Briefly, Australia's health system is a taxpayer-funded national health system which delivers health services through a public health sector and a private health sector. It is a mixed, complex, multi-layered administrative system. There is often a tension between the two sectors as they struggle to achieve a balanced relationship. Services to public patients in public hospitals are free of charge. Medical practitioners employed in public hospitals receive an income as salaried medical officers. Private health practitioners however set their own fees independently of government. Private hospitals are owned and funded by private sector organisations. The public health sector is often the site of funding cutbacks as it is vulnerable to the current policy whims of governments. Funding is often a source of tension between the sectors as the public health sector monitors the extent to which government decides to allocate public funds for public health to the private sector.

Medicare is Australia's universal health insurance scheme which is partly funded by a Medicare levy. The levy is based on taxpayer income level with low-income earners granted an exemption. A Medicare levy surcharge is assigned to high-income earners who have not (as expected) purchased private health insurance. Medicare offers a bulk-billing option, where some medical practitioners elect to receive 85%

of the scheduled fee for service from the government as full payment on behalf of the patient. States and territories have financial responsibilities associated with health across all levels of government with additional funding assistance from the federal government. For example, Queensland health (the system in Queensland) is the overarching body responsible for health at a State level for Queensland. Within each State, medical practitioners are positioned within a medical hierarchy. For example, general medical practitioners (GPs) occupy the lowest position while specialist surgeons occupy the highest positions. This means that specialist surgeons earn more money and attract a higher status than GPs. IMGs however, regardless of their field of practice, tend to be ascribed a lower status by the health system and by Australian trained medical practitioners.

## Foundation of the Study—The Field Work

What might the lived experience of a medical practitioner be like? How would this experience perhaps differ from the lived experience of an internationally trained medical practitioner? IMGs have made and continue to make a significant contribution to rural and remote primary health care. For example, in rural, regional and remote Queensland, the situation reported by Health Workforce Queensland (2011) found that 48.4% of the medical workforce in remote, rural and regional Queensland obtained their basic medical qualifications overseas. In 2015, IMGs still made up just under half (46.9%) of the medical practitioners in remote, rural and regional Queensland. Health Workforce Queensland (2015, p. 9) notes that: "since 2011 the percentage of overseas trained doctors has been relatively stable and has only varied by approximately five per cent". I attended the Australian College of Rural and Remote Medicine (ACRRM) conference in Adelaide. The ACRRM conference assisted me to begin to form some ideas. Two obvious aspects of rural/remote medical practice emerged from conversations and from the conference presentations. Firstly, there was a sense of pride among conference participants. Several presentations highlighted the passion these doctors had for their work as well as their seemingly endless commitment and loyalty to their profession and the communities they served. I felt admiration for them as I listened to some of the ways their commitment was tested. Many faced issues such as small country hospitals struggling to survive, losing services and being under constant threat of closure. Some doctors were located in understaffed practices, worked long hours with minimal access to specialist consultation and other services far away in the cities. Some doctors experienced professional isolation.

It became apparent that rural medicine was framed as less valued than medical practice in cities and metropolitan centres. Conference presentations by several medical practitioners acknowledged that unless one is trained in big city teaching hospitals, one can be considered by those who do practice in these locations, as less qualified. In addition, would be considered as less capable and possibly as having made a poor career decision. Rivett (cited in Gregory et al. 2006, p. 654) confirms:

"There's an intrinsic, inbuilt feeling in a lot of tertiary hospitals that rural practice is not second rate, but even third rate". I considered if the perceived lower status of rural medicine was reason enough to keep some doctors away from taking a rural pathway, therefore contributing to the health workforce shortage in these areas. It was also implied that universities with medical faculties were more inclined to direct teaching and research funding away from rural, remote medicine in favour of mainstream medicine. Moreover, once recruited to rural areas, hospitals experience more difficulty than urban facilities to keep medical staff. This is often due to heavier workloads, with less staff to cover on call rosters and diminished access to specialist services. From their study of nurses working in these areas, Currie et al. (2016, p. 64) concluded: "while GPs continue to provide clinical support in rural areas, they aren't necessarily seen as the essential health care professional". However, Malatzky and Bourke (2016) while accepting that the dominant discourse places rural practice as inferior to urban locations, they challenge the embedded power relations and call for a reframing of rural health to highlight the attractions associated with rural practice. In view of the above, I asked myself if rural medicine is somehow seen as having a lower status, does the fact that many IMGs are required to practice in rural locations mean that IMGs may also be less valued. The next step was to explore against a backdrop of rural practice, the experiences of IMGs particularly, in these settings. To assist me with this, I was able to attend another event, this time an IMG forum organised by the Royal Australian College of General Practitioners (RACGP) (Qld). I attended to listen and observe. Attending the forum was extremely enlightening and several aspects were added to my existing and expanding understanding.

Throughout the three-day forum, I had the opportunity to observe and listen to IMGs who were at various stages in the registration process. There were numerous presentations made and a plethora of information was disseminated to participants. My observations indicated that some doctors were agitated and confused about the processes and associated rules and regulations and many seemed generally overwhelmed. I was not only amazed at how complex the registration process was, but despite the provision of information associated with the process and lengthy explanation, I was also confused. In addition, some doctors seemed annoyed about changes in the system, such as a requirement to resit certain exams.

The personal impact of these stressors became evident when there was a presentation about taking time out, refreshment and renewal in terms of general doctor wellbeing. The presenter sought participation from IMGs regarding how they cared for themselves. A few doctors volunteered their personal experiences and some became emotional while sharing their coping strategies. It was evident that many of the forum participants were generally stressed about their situation and the numerous requirements the system was making of them. This situation seemed to constitute additional pressure to what is commonly regarded as an already stressful occupation.

Every day, medical doctors are required to cope with patient illness, pain and death. In addition, doctors also have to deal with, "A medical-legal and regulatory environment perceived as more threatening, changes to the organisation and funding of health care, and increased accountability of doctors for health outcomes" (Breen et al. 2010 p. xxii). Further, a 2005 study into the psychological health of rural GPs revealed that: "At least one-third to one-half of GPs indicated that they had either 'some degree' or 'quite a lot' of distress directly related to rural general practice" (Gardiner et al. 2005, p. 151). A key finding in the Beyond Blue (2013, p. 2) report on doctor mental health was that: "Doctors reported substantially higher rates of psychological distress than other Australian professions". Medical practice then can be perceived as a generally stressful occupation. A doctor in rural general practice, which appears to be less valued, may be even further stressed due to the conditions of that type of practice. In addition, IMGs in rural or remote locations have a set of other stressors in that they must also negotiate their way through the numerous processes to become registered in Australia.

Ultimately, for this study, I wanted the IMG voice to drive the research. I wanted the participants to raise the aspects of experience which they felt were important in the construction of their experiences and therefore their realities. I began my data collection with a focus group comprised of IMGs.

## The Focus Group

There were six participants (3 men and 3 women). Five of the participants were employed in private practices and one participant was the principal of his own practice. Three broad themes emerged from the one-hour session: *new ways of approaching clinical practice; information and orientation; working conditions.* As the researcher, I wanted the session to flow on their terms with little input from me. The responses given helped focus the research more closely on the experiences of IMG general practitioners in a particular rural community.

Participants made it very clear that the system and its requirements were problematic and several accounts of negative experiences were shared (Pascoe 2011). The system was mentioned extensively throughout the data and was featured especially in the Inquiry submissions. The focus group data gave me a more personalised account and a kind of micro-snapshot of IMG GPs within a particular rural community than the field work experiences. I felt well prepared to progress to the semi-structured interviews. Ten individual semi-structured interviews and submissions to the 2012 Parliamentary Inquiry and 2016 Senate Committee constituted the next stage of data collection.

## The Interviews

The individual interviews afforded me the opportunity to converse with IMGs one to one. Three of the ten were conducted over the phone. The face-to-face interviews were more productive than the phone interviews. Nevertheless, I was glad to be talking with busy medical practitioners on any terms and particularly on their terms. Each interview allowed me into the world of the participant and that was a privilege in itself. The duration of the interviews was around an hour allowing enough time for participants to tell individual stories of lived experience in greater detail. *New Ways of clinical Practice; working conditions; demands of the system* were the emergent themes from the interviews.

The submissions made to a 2012 Parliamentary Inquiry (House of Representatives Standing Committee on Health and Ageing 2012) provided extra voices for my research. The motion for an inquiry was successfully made by Bruce Scott, member for Maranoa on the 18 October 2010. This occurred after much heated parliamentary debate about various aspects related to the treatment of IMGs in Australia by the system. For example, Mr. Scott reported concerns in relation to discrimination in the processes associated with the assessment of IMGs. Mr Scott also raised concerns related to lack of transparency and accuracy within the system and revealed that he knew of IMGs who passed the Royal Australian College of General Practitioners (RACGP) fellowship only to fail their pre-employment structured clinical interview (PESCI). Mr Scott went on to criticise immigration practices at the time which could deport temporary resident IMGs while they awaited the outcome of an appeal. Member of Parliament for Blair Mr. Neuman and Mr. Laming Member of Parliament for Bowman joined the debate and accused the government of ignoring the problem. Mr. Katter Member of Parliament for Kennedy said he knew of cases where IMGs were subjected to "petty vicious and personal vendettas", and Mr. Entsch Member of Parliament for Leichhardt likened the specialist colleges to "the mafia".[1]

As a result of the debate, on Tuesday 23 November 2010, the then Minister for Health and Ageing, the Honourable Nicola Roxon MP, announced that she would task the House of Representatives Standing Committee on Health and Ageing to inquire into and report on *Registration Processes and Support for Overseas Trained Doctors.* I now had representation of the IMG community across Australia to include in my data set. The committee conducted twenty-one public hearings throughout Australia in every State and Territory in twelve different cities. The committee took direct evidence from 145 witnesses during the public hearings. They received 175 submissions from IMGs and interested others from across Australia as well as 22 supplementary submissions. From the total of 216 submissions, 109 were from IMGs and 91 from the various organisations and agencies involved in the registration, regulation, training and support of IMGs. The subsequent findings of the inquiry along with 45 recommendations were produced in a report entitled: "Lost in the Labyrinth".

---

[1] Media Release: Passionate cries in Parliament—"There needs to be fairer go for overseas trained doctors" http://www.connectingup.org/organisation/australian-doctors-trained-overseas-as sociation. Accessed 27 May 2011.

## The 2012 Parliamentary Inquiry on Registration Processes and Support for Overseas Trained Doctors: Submissions

The IMGs, who made submissions, not only included GPs but also contributions from IMGs in other specialist areas. This data was particularly rich as many of the voices wrote heart-felt accounts of personal misadventure and career crisis. Graphic details of bullying and inadequacies in the system led many doctors to the point where they felt the need to inform an inquiry of their experiences. Therefore, the data from the inquiry submissions was primarily negative. The submissions rendered the following key themes: *working conditions; demands of the system; difficulties dealing with the system; bullying; Dr well-being.* The theme of bullying was particularly prominent in the submissions compared with the focus group and interviews (except for one) where there was evidence of bullying practices (in the researcher's opinion) but the practices were not identified directly as "bullying" by the participants. Some of the 2012 inquiry submissions gave graphic examples of bullying and I was shocked that professional adults would exhibit these behaviours, particularly within a perceived esteemed profession. In 2016, I had another opportunity to add to my data set.

On 2 February 2016, the Senate referred the medical complaints process in Australia to the Senate Community Affairs References Committee on Medical Complaints process in Australia, for inquiry and report (The Senate Community Affairs References Committee 2016). Although this inquiry was on a somewhat smaller scale than the 2012 inquiry, it held two public hearings during 2016 (one in Sydney, the other in Canberra) and it received 129 submissions. The impetus for this inquiry came from media exposure of bullying, sexism and sexual harassment within the medical profession, particularly within the surgical specialities. Complaints to the Royal Australasian College of Surgeons led the College to appoint an Expert Advisory Group to investigate (Knowles 2015). The subsequent report revealed a disturbing culture. High-profile Neurosurgeon Dr Charlie Teo, citing adverse personal experiences of this culture (Sherden and Cannane 2015), together with Senators Nick Xenophon and John Madigan successfully lobbied the Senate to establish the 2016 inquiry.

## The 2016 Senate Community Affairs References Committee on Medical Complaints Process in Australia: Submissions

The Committee published additional guidance on the inquiry's terms of reference to clarify that the inquiry's focus was on the intersection between bullying and harassment in Australia's medical profession and the medical complaints process (2016, p. 2). The 2016 inquiry also contained many examples of bullying and harassment. This inquiry gifted me the opportunity to further enhance the strength of the research as I was able to share in not only IMG experiences of bullying but also the stories of affected others within medicine, such as medical students and medical colleagues bullying each other. The submissions to the 2016 inquiry revealed the themes of: *bullying; sexism, sexual harassment, racism, Dr well-being, difficulties dealing with the system and vexatious complaints*. The 2016 Committee noted that a key issue in evidence received was the use of the complaints process as a tool of bullying and harassment to make vexatious complaints (Senate Inquiry 2016, p. 19). What behaviours constitute bullying? There are varying definitions. For example, in their 2016 online survey of bullying, discrimination and sexual harassment for the College of Intensive Care Medicine, Venkatesh et al. (2016, p. 231) defined bullying as:

> The use of force, threat or coercion to abuse, intimidate or aggressively dominate others; systematic and/or continued unwanted and annoying actions of one party or a group, including threats and demands.

Similarly, the 2016 Senate Community Affairs References Committee utilised the definition of bullying offered by the Expert Advisory Panel to the Royal Australasian College of Surgeons (Knowles 2015):

> Bullying is unreasonable and inappropriate behaviour that creates a risk to health and safety. It is behaviour that is repeated over time or occurs as part of a pattern of behaviour. Such behaviour intimidates, offends, degrades, insults or humiliates. It can include psychological, social, and physical bullying. (Appendix 1, p. 19)

In their definition of bullying at work, Matthiesen and Einarsen (2007, p. 735) provide a more formal, academic definition of workplace bullying which importantly mentions the vulnerability of victims in a bullying situation to defend themselves:

> A situation in which one or more persons systematically and over a long period of time perceive themselves to be on the receiving end of negative treatment on the part of one or more persons, in a situation in which the person (s) exposed to the treatment on the part of one or more persons, in a situation in which the person (s) exposed to the treatment has difficulty in defending themselves against this treatment.

There are also various definitions of harassment. A clear definition of harassment offered by Knowles (2015) is:

> Unwanted, unwelcome or uninvited behaviour that makes a person feel humiliated, intimidated or offended. Harassment can include racial hatred and vilification, be related to a disability, or the victimisation of a person who has made a complaint. (Appendix 1, p. 19)

It also became clear from both the 2012 and 2016 Inquires that bullying is a systemic behaviour within medicine itself and for IMGs particularly. Why is there so much controversy surrounding IMGs and their treatment in this country, enough to initiate a Parliamentary Inquiry? The fundamental research question here is: there are medical schools within Australian universities, and from these, Australian trained medical doctors graduate. Why then are there medical doctors from overseas practicing medicine in Australia?

**Table 1** GP workforce numbers by regional grouping and training (Australian or Overseas)

| Years | Major cities | | Regional centres | | Remote centres | |
|---|---|---|---|---|---|---|
| | Australian | Overseas | Australian | Overseas | Australian | Overseas |
| 2000–2001 | 12,902 | 4300 | 3933 | 1534 | 238 | 178 |
| 2008–2009 | 12,649 | 5742 | 4048 | 2670 | 379 | 238 |
| Change | −253 | 1442 | 115 | 1136 | 141 60 | 60 |
| Percentage change (%) | −2.0 | 33.5 | 2.9 | 74.1 | 59.2 | 33.7 |

*Source* Adapted from NRHA, 2011, submission 113, p. 7

# Why Does Australia Need IMGs?

Ultimately Australia is working towards health workforce self-sufficiency. However, Australia will still need the skills of IMGs well into the future. In their submission to the 2012 inquiry, the National Rural Health Alliance (2011) highlighted the fact that in reality, it takes approximately thirteen years for a doctor to become fully qualified. Consequently, IMGs will be needed to assist with the training and supervision of Australian graduates. Dr St (2011, p. 19) informed the Parliamentary Inquiry Committee that it was critical to retain an experienced IMG cohort not only to provide medical services but to also provide clinical oversight of Australian trained health professionals. From his observations, he stated:

> Our foreign doctors are our current teachers, let alone our current providers of care. They teach our local students, our local health workers and our local specialist trainees. So it is more than just the provision of health care.

Table 1 shows the general practice medical doctor workforce trend over a ten-year period.

Why have the numbers of Australian trained GPs declined? The reasons are multi-faceted and according to Rural Health Workforce Australia (2011) include: ageing and subsequent retirement of the GP workforce; inadequate numbers of medical graduates choosing general practice, and of those, fewer still choosing rural practice. Also noted was increasing numbers of GPs wanting to work part-time (particularly women); the lack of appeal of solo practices and overall decline in some rural communities.

As a result, prospective employers of IMGs continue to seek their skills. The House of Representatives' Committee report (2012, p. 18) identified two key issues which were constantly evident in Australia's medical workforce. Firstly, "an inadequate supply of doctors generally" and, secondly, "an uneven geographical distribution of doctors, with workforce shortages remaining acute in some regional areas and particularly in rural and remote locations". This has not always been the case; however, the Australian medical workforce situation has also been perceived as in a state of over-supply. Therefore, government policy over the last two decades has been influenced by concerns of over-supply (1992) to concerns of under-supply (2005) resulting in active recruitment of IMGs (Australian Medical Council 2011).

The Committee of Inquiry into Medical Education and Medical Workforce (1988) advised the Federal Government of the increase in the numbers of IMGs obtaining professional registration and implicated the increase as a significant issue in the subsequent increased outlays nationally via Medicare. In 1992, the Medical Work-force Supply Working Party investigated the supply and requirements of the general practice workforce in Australia and noted a continued trend of over-supply. It was also noted that immigration was the primary influence on the size and shape of the medical workforce. Consequently, the government introduced a number of measures throughout the 1990s in an effort to reduce doctor numbers (Iredale and Gluck 1993). Some of these included a decrease in the number of medical school places and restric-tions on new permanent resident IMGs who successfully gained Australian Medical Council (AMC) accreditation to access Medicare billing for 10 years after regis-tration. There were also various other restrictions on IMG practice if they came to Australia with temporary appointments (Hawthorne and Birrell 2002). According to Dr Haikerwal (2005, p. 5): "The Government got it wrong back in 1996 …They did it at precisely the time we were going into deficit supply. Now we are paying the price". The price has been paid heavily in rural and remote Australia and continues, where communities struggle to recruit medical staff and to retain them. Many people living in these communities as a consequence have to travel long distances to attend the nearest medical care.

By 2003, there was a decline in bulk-billed medical services in regional areas generally and in regional and metropolitan hospitals. Rural communities were in healthcare access crisis because they were unable to recruit doctors. The govern-ment's approach to medical workforce policy shifted to one of medical workforce expansion based on the apparent challenge of too few doctors. Several new medical schools were proposed and financial assistance was introduced for the recruitment of IMGs. Recruitment was especially sought for those IMGs with temporary visas required to work in a sponsored position (Hawthorne and Birrell 2002). Despite these measures, shortages in rural and remote locations persisted.

There has been debate as to the continued reliance on overseas doctors to supple-ment the medical workforce shortage. Some have argued that this trend will be ongo-ing while others believe that the need for IMGs has diminished (see Birrell 2011). The House of Representatives' Committee report (2012, p. 14), however, noted that: "the more widely held view is that there are still too few medical practitioners to meet Australia's needs". Currently, there is no limit to the number of IMGs a sponsor can employ. Recruitment occurs under the permanent-entry employer-sponsorship visa subclass. Organisations can sponsor a doctor trained overseas to work in Australia for up to four years. However, IMGs must gain general registration before a visa is granted.

# The Research Study Underpinning this Book

This study is a qualitative, empirical one which explores the experiences of International Medical Graduates (IMGs) in Australia. The aim is to raise the visibility of IMGs and their experiences by locating them in the centre as a professional community. The objective is to explain why IMGs in reality are positioned as an underclass within Australia's medical dominance. What has been revealed is a power relation struggle. Initially, power is examined through the rise of Medicine and the Medical profession to its position of medical dominance over all other medical/paramedical professions. The power structure bureaucracy created by the Australian health system is referred to as 'the system' which is made up of numerous agencies, bodies and organisations. The system has constructed a complex and confusing set of processes to regulate and control International Medical Graduates as 'the other'. They constitute 'the other' because they are not Australian trained; they have not obtained their basic medical qualification in Australia. I view IMGs as a community of people based on a common professional qualification. While IMGs belong to a high-status profession, the system ensures that IMGs are treated differently than Australian trained doctors and IMGs appear to constitute a community which can be classified as an under-class within the profession. The system communicates with IMGs via a deficit discourse which I argue is underpinned by xenophobia (a fear of things foreign), racism and ethnocentrism (Australian culture is superior to other cultures). Analysis of how IMGs experience Australia utilises an intersectionality framework where the intersecting inequalities of class, race and nation are unpacked. The experiences of IMGs in Australia and the possible foundations for those experiences are explored throughout the following six chapters of this book. This book extends the concept of medical dominance in Australia to focus on the positioning of IMGs within medical dominance. Much of the literature around medical dominance focuses on how medical dominance is created and maintained (see Willlis 1989, 2006; Broome 2006; Germov 2014). The focus of this book is directed towards an understanding of why medical dominance exists. IMGs are medical doctors, as are Australian trained medical doctors, and the medical profession itself constitutes an elite profession. Has the elite profession of medicine become too powerful? A toxic culture has festered and become chronic within medicine itself. A culture of bullying, sexism, sexual harassment and self-interest has become endemic. From colleagues, bullying each other and vexatious complaints made against each other, to the bullying of IMGs and medical students via "pedagogy of humiliation" (Australian Medical Students' Association 2016, Submission 10). It is argued that the medical profession has experienced a power failure, where the source of its implosion has come from within. As such, the obligations of service and care delivery from consummate medical professionals to the Australian public, via a social contract of faith, are questionable (Susskind and Susskind 2015). IMGs that come to Australia come to this environment. Their voices shared throughout the chapters paint a picture of their lived experience in Australia. Other voices shared via the media, the literature and inquiry submissions, enable the reader to not only appreciate IMG experiences, but also other rich narratives of experience which unfold within Australia's dominant medical culture.

## Chapter Overview

Chapter one commences the research presentation and the advancement to establish the positioning of IMGs within Australia's medical culture. Underpinned by a social justice stance and an anti-oppressive approach, methodological decisions and dilemmas are outlined and justified for the reader. As researcher, I identify myself as an Indigenous Australian and my positioning within the research process, that of a scholar writing as a colonised other, an allied other and a Third-World intellectual. Also revealed is my questioning of the suitability for this study of a single-discipline approach and the restrictions which accompany same. I required a model from the heart, one that embraces empathy, emotionality as well as personal accountability (Hill Collins 1991; Hill Collins and Bilge 2016). As a result, a multidisciplinary perspective allows for a more comprehensive and thorough exploration and representation of the IMG voice. In this chapter, the participants are introduced to the reader as well as the recruitment journey and associated challenges. Confidentiality and anonymity are highlighted with particular rigour for these participants, due to the nature of their precarious position and possible repercussions. Post-structural feminism and the concepts of elites and studying up bring useful perspectives to the study. I argue that social justice, anti-oppressive approaches (Strega and Brown 2015) through to the identification of intersecting inequalities to underpin analysis, best facilitate a move towards the explanation of the IMG experience in Australia. Biographies as well as history are fundamental to the investigation of the positioning of IMGs, and in chapter two, a historical lens provides background that sets the scene and flags significant stages. These allow the reader to explore some of the important influences and events that have shaped the Australian nation and its peoples. Discussion traces the journey of Western medicine in Australia from the discovery and subsequent British invasion of the Great Southern Land through to today. The encounters of the newcomers with Australia's Indigenous peoples, the custodians of the land, and their ancient medical practices (Gunstone 2008) are advanced and the first IMGs are introduced. Further discussion progresses through to the arrival of refugee IMGs following the Second World War (Iredale 2009; Kunz 1975) to the current context of medical practice. The emergence of a powerful, high-status medical profession with the ability to successfully lobby governments to further its own agenda becomes evident (Willis et al. 2016). Colonial history shows the development of a fearful xenophobic nation, one which feels threatened by 'others'. Subsequently, IMGs also came to be regarded with suspicion and were eventually ascribed an inferior underclass status. Their credentials and skills were called into question. Chapter two also reveals an ethnocentric and racist Australia where, despite a black Indigenous population, the notion of white supremacy and Western cultural superiority not only flourished but racism was institutionalised in the 1901 Federation of the 'new' nation and the White Australia Policy. The position of status and power afforded to Australian trained medical doctors is perpetuated and reinforced via the development of the Australian nation (Plage et al. 2016) and the intersecting oppressions of class, race and nation. The phenomenon of power and its relationship with IMGs is explored further in chapter three. A matrix of domination facilitates the separation of power into *Structural Power, Hegemonic Power and Interpersonal Power* dimensions (Hill Collins 1990; Hill Collins and Bilge 2016). The power found structurally within the health system and other related organisations which are tasked with the regulation and control of IMGs is further unpacked for the reader. Chapter three provides an outline of the policies and procedures of the system which IMGs must navigate to obtain accreditation and registration in Australia. The IMG voices tell of their experiences in their dealings with the system. The hegemonic power of the medical profession as gatekeepers to the health system is revealed (Willis 1989), and the interpersonal power interaction between IMGs, the system and medical dominance is exposed. Further explanation and exploration of the concept of medical dominance continues into chapter four. Firstly, discussion traces the rise of the medical profession in Australia from the 1870s. Today, Medical dominance wields power over other health professionals in that the medical profession in Australia is the sovereign expert, sanctioned by governments. Medicine's ownership and custodianship of medical knowledge and clinical skills facilitate the profession's expert status. Discussion acknowledges that there are changes in and challenges to medical dominance, but despite its changing nature, medical dominance still manages to evolve as conditions require, while retaining its dominant position (Coburn 2006; Willis 2006). Also revealed in chapter four is the unsavoury side of Australia's medical culture. The toxic culture within the profession has surfaced (particularly since 2015) via the media. Reports of systemic sexism and sexual harassment, bullying, uncompetitive and even unlawful behaviours have been revealed. The surgical specialities were especially exposed initiating the Royal Australasian College of Surgeons to appoint an expert panel to investigate (Knowles 2015). The toxic culture even infiltrates down the hierarchy to medical students prompting the Medical Students' Association to not only speak out against bullying but also to allege that bullying had pushed some medical students to suicide (Campus Review 2015). Here, the reader is invited into the stories of experience from some of those medical professionals, including senior surgeons, who have suffered at the hands of the profession itself. The voices come from the media to join the voices of their colleagues in the IMG community. Chapter five asks the question: "what's the problem with IMGs, is there a problem?" Initially, IMGs as a global resource come into question within a growing climate of the international exchange of ideas, technologies and goods and services. Global conditions have facilitated a migratory workforce and IMGs are in demand.

This leads to an ethical argument in that not only do countries with a medical workforce shortage actively entice and recruit medical doctors from other countries, but they are poached from developing countries to practice in wealthy countries. In opposition to this is the basic human right argument, advancing that a medical doctor should have the freedom to live and work where ever he or she chooses. In addition, medical doctors also move from developed country to developed country such as from the UK to Australia (Dwyer 2007). The reasons behind doctor migration are outlined and include a relocation to experience adventure and life in a new country to those doctors who flee unsafe situations and come as refugees. Medical doctors who leave their country of origin for safety reasons and are unable to return home are rendered vulnerable to the requirements of the Australian system. Perhaps arriving in Australia, already having experienced significant stress could be compounded by the necessity for vulnerable IMGs to place their careers at the mercy of the Australian health system.

Australia's poor human rights record is acknowledged along with idealised perceptions of Australia as an egalitarian country which professes a "fair go for all" (Plage et al. 2016). Further, chapter five notes that IMGs appear to constitute a problem simply because of the numerous inquiries which have been conducted into aspects related to them and their experiences. Organisations that deal with the processes IMGs must navigate through are often criticised with very similar recommendations being made from these inquiries, and very little action being taken. The concept of a wicked problem is introduced in relation to the situation for IMGs in Australia. These problems have a power differential at their core, are multi-causal and have multiple interdependencies. As a result, they are highly resistant to a solution. Following a problem representation approach, Bacchi's (2009) six questions are adapted to scrutinise the problematisation of IMGs. Scrutiny includes revealing, identifying and reflecting on inherent silences within problematisations. For example, in this case the need to maintain the high standard of health care in Australia as justification for discriminatory and unprofessional behaviours towards IMGs. Discussion assists an integrated analysis where the focus is shifted from a problem-solving focus to a problem-questioning focus. Further analysis continues in chapter six where the intersecting inequalities of *class, race* and *nation* are explored. Through the analytic tool of intersectionality, unequal power relations are viewed as intersecting oppressions which conspire together to assign IMGs in Australia an underclass status within the elite profession of Australian medicine. The contribution made to the literature made by this book is consolidated synergistically in chapter six to explain why IMGs are positioned as an underclass. It can be seen how xenophobic, racist and ethnocentric norms, values, assumptions and beliefs have developed to weave their way through Australian society, its governments, its institutions and its laws. The Australian nation influences the socialisation of its peoples, a nation underpinned by a long history of systemic oppressions. In terms of IMGs, the system entrusted with their regulation and control harbours a systemic frustration of aspirations (Eckermann et al. 2006) where medical dominance furthers its own agenda based on self-interest.

This book positions IMGs as a professional community construct and reflects the interconnectedness of the intersections. The intersections of class, race and nation best reflect the positioning of IMGs. Many intersectionality studies include gender as an intersecting oppression but this book has not. While acknowledging that gender is indeed a very important intersection, in this case I did not want to divide the IMG community in any way. Similarly, then ethnicity (also, a much explored intersection in many studies) has not been selected. I sought to empower the IMG community and their voices, not divide them into other categories of IMGs. In this way, as a professional community, IMG solidarity, agency and the associated voices gifted to this study can stand together as one. Chapter six, the final chapter, before concluding also looks more widely for sociopolitical phenomenon. The current emergence and influence of right-wing conservative political platforms are investigated in terms of an angry working class backlash and anti-immigration stance. The political resurrection of Pauline Hanson in Australia, the election of Donald Trump to the presidency of the United States and Britain's vote to exit the European Union, are examples. These events do not represent isolated extremism but rather an underestimated and significant shift of public concerns and fears. A commonality of issues comes to light, those of: the economy, immigration, the maintenance of national identity and a nostalgic return to 'greatness.' Immigration is a primary concern for two reasons, firstly there is fear that migrants take local jobs and secondly migrants are a perceived threat to national identity and security. Muslims are particularly demonised and are often linked to terrorism (Eid 2017; Ewart 2012). Australia's xenophobic stance on immigration and border protection is outlined in this chapter. Australia has a long history of exclusion, and in terms of immigration, the country has moved from suspicion and caution to exclusion to ensure protection from the 'other'. The extraordinary lengths the government will go to keep the 'other' out of Australia, particularly asylum seekers arriving by boat, are unprecedented (Glynn 2016; Higgins 2016; Riley 2016). The 'life-saving' rhetoric around stopping boat arrivals and the image Australia now sends to the world is critiqued in this chapter. Also highlighted is Australia's preoccupation with 'whiteness' (Frankenberg 1993; Knowles 2010) and an ethnocentric belief of superiority (Grigg and Manderson 2016). Australia has always been a racist country, beginning with the massacre and dispossession of Australia's first peoples. The Australian nation's obsession with whiteness is perpetuated today through Australia's institutions and policies where racism has been institutionalised and Indigenous Australians remain marginalised (see Gunstone 2017). For IMGs who come to Australia, what does our society reflect back to them and how do they retain their professional identity as medical doctors amidst the questioning of their credentials? (Harris and Guillemin 2015). Some IMGs never have their credentials accredited and join the medical unemployed while others may find themselves in exploitative workplaces where they experience bullying and discrimination (Knowles 2015; Venkatesh et al. 2016). The focus of this book is on the IMG experience, and the voices woven throughout the following chapters reveal those experiences. Analysis concludes that IMGs in Australia are positioned as an underclass within the elite profession of medicine.

# References

Bacchi, C. (2009). *Analysing policy: What's the problem represented to be?*. Frenchs Forest NSW: Pearson Australia.
Beyond Blue. (2013). *National mental health survey of doctors and medical students.* Viewed 12 October 2015, www.beyondblue.org.au.

Birrell, B. (2011). *Australia's new health crisis—Too many doctors*. Viewed 27 January 2012, http://arts.monash.edu.au/cpur/–downloads/australias-new-health-crisis.pdf.

Breen, K. J., Cordner, S. M., Thomson, C. J. H., & Plueckhahn, V. D. (2010). *Good medical practice: Professionalism, ethics and law*. New York: Cambridge University Press.

Broom, A. (2006). Reflections on the centrality of power in medical sociology: An empirical test and theoretical elaboration. *Health Sociology Review, 15*(5), 496–505.

Campus Review. (2015). *Students want change of medical culture*. Campus Review. Viewed 12 March 2016, https://www.campusreview.com.au.

Coburn, D. (2006). Medical dominance then and now: Critical reflections. *Health Sociology Review, 15*(5), 432–443.

Committee of Inquiry into Medical Education and Medical Workforce. (1988). *Australian Medical Education and Workforce into the 21st century*, Canberra.

Currie, F., Nielsen, G., & Ervin, K. (2016). The value of rural isolated practice endorsed registered nurses in a small rural health service. *Research in Health Science, 1*(1), 58–67. Viewed 9 January 2017, http://www.scholink.org/ojs/index.php/rhs.

Dwyer, J. (2007). What's wrong with the global migration of health care professionals? Individual rights and international justice. *Hastings Center Report, 37*(5), 36–43.

Eckermann, A. K., Dowd, T., Chong, E., Nixon, L., Gray, R., & Johnson, S. (2006). *Binan Goonj: Bridging cultures in Aboriginal health* (2nd ed.). Marrickville: Churchill Livingstone Elsevier.

Eid, M. (2017). Ethics, decision-making, and risk communication in the Era of Terroredia: The case of ISIL. In *Violence and society: Breakthroughs in research and practice*. University of Ottawa, Canada.

Ewart, J. (2012). Framing an alleged terrorist: How four Australian news media organisations framed the Dr. Mohamed Haneef case. *Journal of Media and Religion, 11*(2), 91–106.

Frankenberg, R. (1993). *White women, race matters: The social construction of whiteness*. London, New York: Routledge.

Gardiner, M., Sexton, R., Durbridge, M., & Garrard, K. (2005). The role of psychological well-being in retaining rural general practitioners. *Australian Journal of Rural Health, 13,* 149–155.

Germov, (Ed.). (2014). *Second opinion* (5th ed.). South Melbourne, Australia: Oxford University Press.

Glynn, I. (2016). *Asylum policy, boat people and political discourse: Boats, votes and asylum in Australia and Italy*. UK: Palgrave Macmillan, viewed 8 November 2016, via Springer link (Flinders university) http://download.springer.com.exyproxy.

Gregory, A., Armstrong, R., & Van Der Weyden, M. (2006). Rural and remote health in Australia: How to avert the deepening health care drought. *Medical Journal of Australia, 185*(11/12), 654–660.

Grigg, K., & Manderson, L. (2016). The Australian racism, acceptance, and cultural—Ethnocentrism scale (RACES): Item response theory findings. *International Journal for Equity in Health, 15*(49), 1–16, viewed 9 March 2017, https://doi.org/10.1186/s12939-016-0338-4, http://equityhealthj.biomedcentral.com/articles/10.1186/s.

Gunstone, (Ed.). (2008). *History, politics and knowledge: Essays in Australian Indigenous studies*. Melbourne VIC: Australian Scholarly Publishing Pty Ltd.

Gunstone, (2017). Reconciliation, peacebuilding and indigenous people in Australia. In H. Devere, K. Te Maiharoa, & J. P. Synott (Eds.), *Peacebuilding and the rights of indigenous people: Experiences and strategies for the 21st century* (pp. 17–28). Berlin: Springer.

Haikerwal, M. (2005). *Observations from an overseas trained doctor*. Australian Medical Association, viewed 5 April 2007, http://www.ama.com.au/web.nsf/doc/WEEN-6EG7CN.

Harris, A., & Guillemin, M. (2015). Notes on the medical underground: Migrant doctors at the margins. *Health Sociology Review, 24*(2), 163–174. https://doi.org/10.1080/14461242.2014.999403.

Hawthorne, L., & Birrell, B. (2002). Doctor shortages and their impact on the quality of medical care in Australia. *People and Place, 10*(3), 55–67.

Health Workforce Queensland. (2011). *Medical practice in rural and remote Queensland: Minimum data set*. Brisbane: Health Workforce Queensland.

Health Workforce Queensland. (2015). *A snapshot of the health workforce landscape in Queensland*. Brisbane: Health workforce Queensland.

Higgins, C. (2016). Status determination of Indochinese boat arrivals: A 'balancing act' in Australia. *Journal of Refugee Studies*, 1–17. Viewed 19 December 2016, https://doi.org/10.1093/jrs/fev036, (Downloaded at Flinders University of South Australia) http://jrs.oxfordjournals.org/.

Hill Collins, P., & Bilge, S. (2016). *Intersectionality*. Cambridge, UK: Polity press.

Hill Collins, P. (1990). *Black feminist thought: Knowledge, consciousness, and the politics of empowerment, perspectives on gender* (Vol. 2). Boston: Unwin Hyman.

Hill Collins, P. (1991). *Black feminist thought: Knowledge, consciousness, and the politics of empowerment*. Boston MA: Unwin Hyman.

House of Representatives Standing Committee on Health and Ageing. (2012). *Lost in the Labyrinth: Report on the inquiry into registration processes and support for overseas trained doctors*. Canberra: The Parliament of the Commonwealth of Australia.

Iredale. (2009). Luring overseas trained doctors to Australia: Issues of training, regulating and trading. *International Migration, 47*(4), 31–64.

Iredale, R., & Gluck, M. (1993). The medical quota. *Health professionals in multicultural Australia*, 16–34.

Keim, T., Vogler, S., Tin, J., & Baskin, B. (2013) Dr Death gets off: Manslaughter charges dropped against Jayant Patel, LNP and Labor start blame game. *Courier Mail*, 16 November.

Knowles, C. (2010). Theorising race and ethnicity: Contemporary paradigms and perspectives. In P. Hill Collins & J. Solomos (Eds.), *The Sage handbook of race and ethnic studies* (pp. 23–42). London: Sage Publications.

Knowles, R. (2015). *Expert advisory group draft report on discrimination, bullying and sexual harassment*. Melbourne: Royal Australasian College of Surgeons. https://www.surgeons.org/media/22045685eag-report-to-racs-draft-08-sept-2015.pdf.

Kunz, E. F. (1975). *The intruders: Refugee doctors in Australia*. Canberra: Australian national University Press.

Malatzky, C., & Bourke, L. (2016). Re-producing rural health: Challenging dominant discourses and the manifestation of power. *Journal of Rural Studies, 45,* 157–164.

Matthiesen, S., & Einarsen, S. (2007). Perpetrators and targets of bullying at work: Role, stress and individual differences. *Violence and Victim, 22*(6), 735–753.

Pascoe. (2011). *Experiences of culture shock, vulnerability and powerlessness: Reflections from international medical graduates and the impact on their wellbeing*. Paper presented to 2011 Migration update South Australia and beyond, Adelaide, 23–24 June 2011.

Plage, S., Willing, I., Skrbis, Z., & Woodward, I. (2016). Australiannes as fairness: Implications for cosmopolitan encounters. *Journal of Sociology, 1*(6), 1–16, viewed 9 February 2017, via Sage (Flinders University, South Australia) http://jos.sagepub.com.

Riley, A. (2016). Same old rhetoric cannot justify banning refugees from Australia. *The Conversation*, viewed 17 November 2016, http://www.theconversation.com/same-old-rhetoric-cannot-justify-banning-refugees-from-australia-67923.

Rural Health Workforce. (2011). Viewed 14 June 2011, http://www.rhwa.org.au/site/index.cfm?display=120153.

Sherden, A. & Cannane, S. (2015). *Neurosurgeon Dr Charlie Teo says 'bullying culture' in medicine destroying lives, backs call for inquiry* . Lateline 4 September 2015, http://www.abc.net.au/lateline.

Strega, S., & Brown, L. (Eds.). (2015). *Research as resistance: Revisiting critical, indigenous, and anti-oppressive approaches*. Toronto: Canadian scholar's press.

Susskind, R., & Susskind, D. (2015). *The future of the professions: How technology will transform the work of human experts*. New York: Oxford University Press.

The Senate Community Affairs References Committee. (2016). *Medical complaints process in Australia*, Canberra.

Tulloch, J., & Lupton, D. (2003). *Risk and everyday life*. London: Sage publications.

Venkatesh, B., Corke, C., Raper, R., Pinder, M., Stephens, D., Joynt, G., et al. (2016). Prevalence of bullying, discrimination and sexual harassment among trainees and fellows of the college of intensive care medicine of Australia and New Zealand. *Critical Care and Resuscitation, 18*(4), 230–234.

Willis, E. (1989) *Medical dominance: The division of labour in Australian health care*, revised edn. North Sydney: Allen & Unwin.

Willis, E. (2006). Introduction: Taking stock of medical dominance. *Health Sociology Review, 15*(5), 421–431.

Willis, E., Reynolds, L., & Keleher, H. (Eds.). (2016). *Understanding the Australian health care system* (3rd ed.). Chatswood, NSW: Elsevier.

# The Pathway to Find the Voices

Qualitative researchers are guests in the private spaces of the world. Their manners should be good and their code of ethics strict (Stake 2000, p. 447).

It is fruitful to think that all research must be reflexive and that in many ways the researchers should treat all the researched…as elites (Tomic and Trumper 2012, p. 244).

## Introduction

The exploration of how IMGs perceive and experience their realities working and living in Australian communities represents a qualitative, empirical study. The most suitable approach to the overarching research question: "How are IMGs positioned within Australia's medical culture" was to adopt a multidisciplinary view. This decision was taken to avoid the constraints of discipline boundaries, which in turn, can potentially limit the breadth of explanation in answer to the question. Subsequently, this position supports the social justice, anti-oppressive approach taken. In this chapter, my research position in terms of who I am in this process will be outlined, from my initial explorations through to putting the research processes in place. My rationale for these methods and their strengths and weaknesses will also be outlined as well as how I moved through the process of data collection. In this chapter, the participants of this study are introduced to the reader. In addition, ethical considerations in relation to the study will be raised and discussed. Theoretical frameworks which resonate with me are also introduced. Post-structural feminism and the concepts of elites and studying up bring useful perspectives to the study. I argue that social justice, anti-oppressive approaches (Strega 2015) through to the identification of intersecting inequalities to underpin analysis, best facilitate a move towards the explanation of the IMG experience in Australia.

© Springer Nature Singapore Pte Ltd. 2019
V. A. Pascoe, *Australia's Toxic Medical Culture*,
https://doi.org/10.1007/978-981-13-2426-0_2

## My Perspective as Researcher

Where do I stand in all this? Who am I? I am the researcher for this study, but I am also an Indigenous Australian, seeking the voices of IMGs who have come from other countries to live and work in Australia. A fundamental requirement of Indigenous research methodology is the identity and location of the voice of the researcher; therefore, I position myself at the outset. I am an Arrernte woman. My Indigenous ancestry comes from my paternal side; this is my position. As Absolon and Willett (2005, p. 97) confirm:

> the location from which the voice of the researcher emanates is an Aboriginal way of ensuring that those who study, write, and participate in knowledge creation are accountable for their own positionality.

This is a way to validate myself and my location within the research process itself. I bring to the research my own collection of experiences and feelings, which construct the many epistemological lenses I look through. Most importantly, "The sociologist requires a sensitivity to and a curiosity about both what is visible and what is not visible to immediate perception and sufficient self-understanding to make possible an empathy with the roles and values of others" (Vidich and Lyman 2003, p. 55). Observations via my fieldwork, during the focus group and subsequent interviews reflected the situation of IMGs as being 'othered'. In addition, the submissions to the 2012 Parliamentary Inquiry and the 2016 Senate Inquiry overwhelmingly endorsed this position. This is not in terms of the simple research process of the researcher and the researched (the other). Rather, I am referring to marginalisation where the dominant culture constructs and maintains rules for regulating social action. "Dominant perspectives distort the realities of the other in an effort to maintain power relations that continue to disadvantage those who are locked out of the mainstream" (Ladson-Billings 2003, p. 408). As an Indigenous Australian scholar, I write as the colonised, another other or an "allied other" (Kaomea 2004, p. 4). Indigenous Australians are marginalised by the dominant culture in this country. Commenting on her social justice work, Hill Collins (2013, p. 67) argues that a researcher located in the margins can access a creative tension:

> They develop a critical consciousness of the need to remain attentive to the connections linking their scholarship and their in-between status of belonging, yet not belonging.

Similarly, the participants in this research constitute a marginalised group. What is particularly interesting in this case is that while IMGs are essentially an elite group in that they are medical practitioners, and at the same time, they are a marginalised group because they are treated by the health system as the other, a different discrete group of people who are not members of the Australian trained medical group. How can I situate myself in this context? I am able to emphasise with the other because my people have experienced the category of other since 1788 until today and will into the future.[1] I have a heightened awareness not only of what it is like to be categorised as other but also of the ramifications, and how they play out over time, for those who are categorised as other.

I am, however, also familiar with the Western way, the dominant way of knowing and doing in higher education. I was raised in the Western way by adoptive Western parents, look Western (to most Westerners) and have Western ancestry. Am I then a 'post-colonial' intellectual? Perhaps I am a Third World intellectual or a 'flash black'.[2] What is ethically important here is for me to declare my position and to have it noted by the reader. This disclosure, however, as highlighted by Maori academic Linda Tuhiwai Smith, can constitute a risk for the researcher's work as Third World intellectuals may have their work undervalued. "Third World intellectuals have to position themselves strategically as intellectuals within the academy, within the Third World or Indigenous world, and within the Western world in which many intellectuals actually work…Their place in the academy is still highly problematic" (Smith 1999, p. 71). I have a lived experience within the academy and I have a lived experience as an Indigenous Australian woman. I also have a lived experience of my other side, within the Western world in which I was raised.

Ultimately, I did not see my empathic relationship with the other and marginalised groups as problematic within this study:

> Although it is true that at some level all research is a uniquely individual enterprise-not part of a sacrosanct body of accumulating knowledge-it is also true that it is always guided by values that are not unique to the investigator: We are all creatures of our own social and cultural pasts (Vidich and Lyman 2003, p. 95).

Critical reflection, while important, should not become the focus or purpose of the research as Strega (2015, p. 146) reminds: "Our positionalities as researchers must be noticed, questioned, and taken up, …: the reader must still learn more about the puzzle or experience being analysed than about the researcher". In fact, empathy is an important tool for understanding the lived experience of others and becomes part of the research process when embodiment is key to the research (Magnat 2012). As the researcher's position in this study is now declared, two important concepts come to light when establishing the position of IMGs in this study: firstly the idea of researching elites and secondly the concept of studying up. The profession of medicine attracts high status and prestige across the globe and can be perceived as an elite profession. As a result, given my position (an Indigenous Australian academic seeking to interview medical doctors), I was in fact studying up. However, while IMGs belong to the elite profession of medicine, they are not granted full acceptance, equality and inclusion into the Australian trained medical doctors' exclusive status. Conversely then, rather than enjoying the same status as their Australian trained colleagues, IMGs, while still a part of the medical profession, can be relegated to an

---

[1]This is clearly demonstrated, for example, in the government's Stronger Futures legislation which continues the Northern Territory Emergency Response. As a result, Indigenous communities in the Northern Territory remain under punitive federal controls (Roffee 2016).
[2]The term 'flash black' is sometimes used to refer to Indigenous Australians with a university education and/or high-paying occupation.

underclass within an elite class. IMGs unable to have their qualifications recognised or awaiting recognition of their qualifications in Australia can be found driving taxis and delivering pizza (Pascoe 2011). Similarly, a participating doctor in a study exploring the retention of IMGs in Victoria conducted by Hawthorne et al. (2004, p. 14) revealed:

> I was approved by Australian government as refugee and they shifted me here. I was quite shocked initially. I showed them my papers and they said they don't care... For a couple of years I was out of job, on unemployment benefits. It was shocking. You can't imagine really, having some type of status, even coming from communist country as refugee and suddenly being nobody. On the other hand I had to get some money for my family. I did four or five different jobs, from taxi driver to building industry to painting things like that.

Perhaps this paradox indicates that I was also studying down?

## Elites and Studying up; or Perhaps Down?

Qualitative research on elites is scarce which led Savage and Williams to entitle their book "Remembering Elites" (Savage and Williams 2008). They argue that apart from the post-war work of Mills (1956) who positioned elites in the economy, the military and the political arenas, there is little research on elites in contemporary sociology compared to classical sociology which was founded on elites and social change. The historical focus on elites began to fade in the early 1970s due to case study research being subjugated by the scientific method of the sample survey. This was a time when researchers began to abandon interviewing elites due to time constraints and access problems (Savage and Williams 2008).

Can an elite be defined? Who is elite? The search for a definition of what constitutes an elite is problematic and ongoing. Hiller (1996), for example, views contemporary elites as small highly organised and integrated groups which exhibit solidarity and cohesion. Pakulski (2011, pp. 329–330) believes that there can be internal divisions within a group of elites but their cohesiveness nurtures "communication, collaboration and collusion, especially the formation of extensive networks". Historically, elite as a concept has changing meanings and moving boundaries. The contemporary view is still illusive therefore: "Elite is a fuzzy concept. From a post-structural approach elites need to be considered flexibly" (Tomic and Trumper 2012, p. 248). I agree with this given my position as researcher and the somewhat dual position (members of an elite profession but an underclass within that profession) of the participants in this study. The participants, while belonging to an elite profession, did not fit the images that come to mind when one thinks of elites, such as the super wealthy, celebrity, business tycoon or royalty perhaps. The participants in no way displayed an elite status, and I did not feel inferior or intimidated at any time during the focus group session or during interviews (face-to-face or via telephone).

Brenda Beagan, A Canadian University of British Columbia (UBC) doctoral student, in 1999 interviewed medical faculty doctors and medical students at UBC.

As a female graduate student, her income and power was much less than the faculty medical doctors she was interviewing. Many of the participating doctors treated her and her research with disrespect and dismissiveness. In contrast, she found that interviewing medical students who were fellow UBC students was a more pleasant undertaking where her relationship seemed to be perceived as on the same level as the participants. Tomic and Trumper (2012, p. 244) make comment on the status of medical doctors in Canada: "Medical doctors are notorious in North America for their social status, income, and a culture of superiority, unparalleled by other professions, a position actively cultivated by physicians". The data from this study and other relevant literature (see Willis et al. 2016) indicates that Australian trained medical doctors are positioned at a similar level to that of their Canadian colleagues.

During my fieldwork, I had the opportunity to observe, take notes and listen. These strategies are particularly helpful for infiltrating elite groups. Ortner (2010, p. 213) refers to this as "interface ethnography". In her discussion of the concept of productive disorientation, Magnat (2012, p. 183) likens fieldwork to a form of "psycho-physical displacement" where fieldwork requires the researcher to abandon control of any research questions and any ideas about the way fieldwork should be conducted and become "displaced, transported and affected". The research *design* was established following an interpretive approach as I was seeking thick description and analysis to understand meaning.

## Design of the Study

As a qualitative researcher, I needed to begin the research encounter with humbling myself to the kind of humility where the researcher lets go of what is known. This state of mind that encourages the researcher to surrender to the openness and wonder of inquiry is suggested by Vagle (2014, p. 15): "It is the kind of humility we engage when we try to stop being so certain of what we know and think. It is the kind of humility evinced when we truly consider new things. It is the type of humility in which we let go". This stance allowed me as researcher and writer the scope to humbly reconstruct life experience where meanings resonate together with reflexivity. I did not seek to work towards finding more accurate ways to explain how something works. Rather, I sought to question, explore and expose how things are experienced by groups of people doing what they do as they live in the world. I sought to build the story from my first-hand observations and the lived experience of participants. Transcripts and the submissions to the Parliament Inquiry (2012) and the Senate Inquiry (2016) were read and reread many times as was my report from the focus group session (Pascoe 2007). I also listened and relistened to the interview recordings. I was acutely aware that sensitively and respectfully representing the gifted voices of participants and their lived experience cannot be merely reduced to a process. The voices became so much more than just data to be clustered, categorised, analysed and reported.

Three major overarching themes emerged from my engagement with and analysis of the data: *class, race* and *nation.* Analysis of the data showed that the intersection of *class, race* and *nation* assisted and collaborated to create and influence the participating IMG experience in Australia. Intersectionality, a feminist emancipatory theoretical framework initially developed by critical race scholar, Crenshaw (1991), became a useful analytic tool to highlight the intersecting inequalities found in IMG narratives against a background of structure and agency. The matrix of domination work of Hill Collins (1991) was helpful in the conceptualisation of a power differential.

## The Participants and Recruitment

None of the IMGs who participated in this study had English as their first language. Two focus group participants (males) and five interview participants (three males and two females) had left their country of origin and come to practise in Australia via another country.

Elite groups (such as medical practitioners) are often difficult to access. Although they tend to be visible and relatively easy to find, they have the ability to put up barriers and refuse access to researchers (Hertz and Imber 1993). I was determined to not be discouraged by recruitment difficulties and took the following advice: "Obstacles to access are challenging but should not provide an excuse to avoid committing to and persevering in studying up" (Aguiar 2012, p. 9). The very nature of the medical profession made scheduling problematic. In some cases, interviews were postponed due to unforeseen circumstances such as patient emergencies. In addition, three doctors consented to be interviewed only via telephone, instead of face-to-face. Snowball sampling is a non-probability strategy which is particularly useful to access difficult-to-penetrate population groups. Berg (2004) explains: "In many instances, researchers conduct studies in areas in which they simply do not know anyone who can serve as the kind of entrance guide or core to a snowball sample to be rolled through the project..." I was grateful when an interview was organised and even more grateful when it actually took place. I very quickly realised that I had to make the best of every situation even when the situation was not ideal. Data collection in terms of the focus group was far less complicated than organising the interviews as the recruitment and preparation had been done for me by the staff of the Division of General Practice.

As the researcher, it was my role to make sure, to the best of my ability, that participants felt protected and empowered throughout the research process. I also needed to ensure that participant information and contributions to the research remained confidential.

# Confidentiality

The participants in this research represented a somewhat fragile group. Many IMGs were currently experiencing or had in the past experienced adverse interactions with various bodies in the Australian Health System responsible for their registration and its associated processes. Some IMGs initiated complaints and appeals associated with their experiences of the processes. Moreover, some IMGs will not speak out against perceived unfair or unreasonable treatment because they fear that their transition through the processes may be jeopardised as a result of making a fuss or going public. This was also evident in the responses to the 2012 Parliamentary Inquiry, where one-third of IMGs requested anonymity (House of Representatives Standing Committee on Health and Ageing 2012, p. x). The Senate Community Affairs References Committee of 2016 took anonymity further and determined that all submissions made by individual medical practitioners that detailed personal experiences of bullying were to be received in confidence (The Senate Community Affairs References Committee 2016, p. 11). These submissions were made unavailable due to the sensitive nature of the content (experiences of bullying) and the possibility that some experiences could be currently under investigation.

Similarly, the expert advisory group to the RACS (Knowles 2015, p. 5) reported that a culture of: "fear and reprisal stopped some Fellows, Trainees and IMGs participating in the research and consultation processes". It is also important to bear in mind that some IMGs come from countries where there is political instability, unrest, violence and corruption. Perhaps as a result, they could feel apprehensive about what may happen to them or even their families because of the information they offered to this research. For example, one of the participants in this study, Shaun (2012, interview 8) when criticising the system during our interview, said: "In my country I could get arrested for this". He then laughed, but this did not detract from the seriousness of the statement. This doctor also mentioned that he had contributed an article which was somewhat critical of his country to an overseas magazine. The article was written in Spanish, not in his first language. Somehow, the article found its way to his home country in the Middle East and a tense time followed as some of his family members still in his home country were questioned by authorities.

I adopted several strategies. Firstly, in terms of confidentiality, I was the only person to interview participants, and although I received some assistance with interview transcription, the electronic files sent for transcription did not have identifying information. In terms of the focus group however, the identity of the IMGs who attended was known to the staff of the division. I was the only one to analyse the data collected at the session however, and the report I produced for the division did not attribute any comments to a particular participant.

## Anonymity

Participating doctors were assured of anonymity and were assigned a pseudonym. However, I discovered that there are very small numbers of IMGs from particular countries practising in Australia. Some rural and remote communities only have one doctor and some only have IMGs. Therefore, the exact location of a doctor and his or her country of origin could be sufficient information to identify the participant. As a result, this book will also not reveal participants' location in Australia. I have endeavoured to select pseudonyms which do not imply a country of origin or cultural/religious affiliation. The voices included in this research selected from the submissions to the 2012 Parliamentary Inquiry and the 2016 Senate Inquiry however, where the doctor did not request to remain anonymous, retain the name of the doctor concerned, represented in initial form only. Even though these particular doctors expressly gave the committees in writing, permission to publish their names, I was aware that the doctor may not wish to have their name mentioned within the context of a book. The submissions to the 2012 inquiry were publically available on the inquiry's website. In terms of the submissions to the 2016 inquiry, as already noted, some were not accessible and these were clearly marked on the 2016 inquiry's website. The submissions available and utilised from the 2016 inquiry then were made by doctors who did not give graphic detail of actual experiences but perhaps outlined how they were feeling about their experiences and the impact of those experiences. My first data collection experience in this study was via the focus group. According to Krueger (1994), the purpose of focus groups is to produce qualitative data that gives insight into attitudes, opinions and perceptions of participants.

## The Focus Group

I was invited by the CEO of a Division of General Practice to facilitate a focus group of IMGs and provide the division with a report on the findings (Pascoe 2007). Six doctors took part, three men and three women. At the time of the session, all participants were currently employed in general practice in a rural community in Queensland. The focus group provided local IMGs with an opportunity to raise and discuss aspects which were integral to their professional and personal lives. Focus groups can facilitate access to the "natural" interaction between and among participants. According to Kamberelis and Dimitriadis (2008, p. 389), focus groups privilege "horizontal interaction" over "vertical interaction" and become social spaces that tend to decrease the influence of the researcher in controlling the topics and flow of interaction". Gilding (2010) suggests that elites may be psychologically motivated to participate in research for the opportunity of personal therapy and self-reflection.

The focus group was unstructured allowing IMGs to freely raise and discuss any aspects they wished. In the invitation distributed to members, the division listed the following as prompts for discussion:

- What assistance do you need as an IMG?
- How can general practices and this division make the transition to Australia easier for IMGs?
- How can we put these ideas into practice?

Initially, as an icebreaker, I asked the participating doctors *why they had chosen to relocate to Australia?* Overwhelmingly, the primary reason was to live and raise a family in a relatively safe country where one's children had access to a reasonable education from an English-speaking background. They did not relocate because they considered employment and living conditions more lucrative or attractive in Australia. This proved to be an effective beginning for our discussion. Ultimately, participants sought and valued safety above everything else. Two focus group participants mentioned that they had come to Australia via South Africa, a country other than their country of origin. Both doctors considered South Africa to be a very lucrative destination for IMGs, more so than Australia, but they also considered it to be unsafe.

One of the doctors stated:

In South Africa we were treated like gods, we had everything. But it is not safe there (Pascoe 2007).

Participating IMGs raised several issues which they viewed as vital to improve the transition of IMGs into the Australian medical workforce. These issues included: orientation, access to information, mentoring and supervision. In addition, certain aspects of personal experience richly illustrated the frustrations, disappointments and difficulties faced by these doctors. These aspects included: working conditions, different cultural perceptions and beliefs, different rules and responsibilities in medical practice and feelings of powerlessness and vulnerability.

The retention rate in general of IMGs in rural and remote Australia is poor. The Australian Rural and Remote Workforce Agencies Group (ARRWAG) (2005, p. 13) in its submission to the 2005 Productivity Commission on Health Workforce identified the following barriers to retaining IMGs and their families in rural Australia:

- poor language skills;
- lack of employment for partners;
- limited educational opportunities for children;
- long working hours and difficulties in providing locum cover;
- religious, cultural or social needs that cannot be accommodated in a small community;
- isolation from cultural networks that may exist elsewhere in the country;
- long distance to travel—particularly for those coming from countries with smaller geographical distances;
- lack of training and orientation in rural medicine;
- difficulties in obtaining support from other medical professionals;
- personality types that find social isolation difficult to deal with.

In terms of the focus group session, the data is broadly grouped under the three following themes: *New ways of approaching clinical practice; information and orientation; and working conditions.*

## New Ways of Approaching Clinical Practice

The practice of medicine varies internationally. Australia has its own medical culture; one doctor stated:

> Every country is different, it's all very different and all very new and that seems to be something you have to learn along the way (Pascoe 2007).

Two participants who previously spent time working in hospital settings in South Africa mentioned several differences between practice in South Africa and Australia. For example, working in emergency in Australia usually does not involve many patients presenting with stab and gunshot wounds as is the case in South Africa. One of the doctors made the point that IMGs from other countries may be more used to dealing with infectious diseases such as HIV, rather than geriatric-related problems and skin cancers which are more common in Australia. The other participant who had spent time working in South Africa stated:

> My first time in emergency here, there was a sprained ankle and a baby with a fever, I thought where's the emergency? (Pascoe 2007).

This doctor also referred to different requirements in his general practice surgery while residing in South Africa:

> In my surgery in South Africa, I could do an aspiration full tracheotomy, whereas in Australia you do it in a hospital because one of the requirements is to have emergency resuscitation equipment. These things are very important to know (Pascoe 2007).

Also raised were different cultural perceptions on 'appropriate care'. The Australian perception of appropriate medical care can also be quite different than the IMG cultural perception. For example, one participant stated:

> I come across patients who would demand the maximum in any situation...we go overboard trying to save lives here (Pascoe 2007).

Participants stressed the importance of assisting IMGs who practise in Australia to be aware of differences. Australian culture requires an IMG to put aside his or her philosophy and beliefs and think and practise in the Australian way. Another doctor gave an example:

> I personally don't believe in the morning after pill but I prescribe it. My values and beliefs are for myself not for the other person (Pascoe 2007).

This part of the discussion led another participant to raise the possibility of litigation in Australia, an action virtually unheard of in his country of origin.

For me to accept death for example, it's very easy because when it's time it happens and that's finished. In my culture litigation would be unheard of because when the time comes it comes. The approach here is so different (Pascoe 2007).

It was agreed generally that awareness of Australian cultural norms, values and beliefs need to be formalised in training. Cultural norms cannot be readily picked up in conversations with colleagues because as one participant mentioned: "Most doctors just do not have time for these conversations" (Pascoe 2007).

It was also noted, however, that access to training was difficult due to distance and finding available time. Most training was held in Brisbane over weekends and this was not a preferred option. One participant also raised the fact that in Australia, there are more drugs available for doctors to prescribe than in many other countries. This doctor commented:

Some mentoring would be particularly helpful in drug identification, prescription and management, there are so many drugs here (Pascoe 2007).

This statement moved the discussion to aspects of mentoring generally and a specific example of one doctor mentoring another. While mentoring IMGs is not a formal requirement, there is mentor training available for doctors who wish to become mentors. It was mentioned that some general practices in the area were keen to mentor IMGs, but did not due to the high turnover rate. Some participants felt that mentoring did have the potential to be formalised; one participant stated:

There needs to be specific guidelines about mentoring where the roles and responsibilities of all parties are clearly set out…but the guidelines need to have flexibility to accommodate different levels of need (Pascoe 2007).

Another participant was currently mentoring a colleague and explained at length:

She had this set back because she had just come to Australia, got a job as a GP out in the bush by herself, with no support services. She is seeking visiting rights to the local hospital in another country town so she is currently not able to care for her patients when they are hospitalised. To get that access she is required to enrol with one of the colleges and take on mentoring (Pascoe 2007).

The mentoring doctor visits her practice and, with patient permission, sits in on consultations. The mentor discusses the cases with the mentee and assesses how she relates to the staff. While this is an extra workload for the mentor, he acknowledged that: "Someone has to do it" (Pascoe 2007). The mentoring doctor has not undertaken formal mentoring training. Instead, he prefers to mentor from his own personal experience:

Whilst I was new in Australia and working towards my FRACGP,[3] I mentally made a note of all that I would have liked assistance with. I didn't need to be taught all over again but just the local practice of medicine. I provide that to a person now and she feels comfortable getting it from me because, probably I'm an IMG. We both feel more comfortable with me telling her what to do and maybe that's a cultural thing (Pascoe 2007).

---

[3] Fellow of the Royal Australian College of General Practitioners.

Mentoring while a time-consuming activity was seen as providing essential advice and support to fellow IMGs. All participants indicated that they would not only be interested in mentoring but they would also be grateful to receive mentoring.

Another doctor voiced legal concerns in relation to mentoring:

> Some doctors have the notion that if you are mentoring someone and that person stuffs up, does the mentor have indemnity? This is a very important issue that needs to be clear. Medical insurance needs to clarify that you may be mentoring but you are not taking that responsibility (Pascoe 2007).

It seemed that the participants wanted more information in order to be informed about what is required in Australia not just in terms of the practice of medicine but also in terms of general knowledge.

## Information and Orientation

While it was acknowledged that there is general information available, participants were seeking more localised information. General information about living and working in Australia is useful but one doctor stated:

> There is no booklet out there that you receive the day you arrive in Australia which says: If you need this… (Pascoe 2007).

Participants stated that easy access to local knowledge was vital, as there are numerous situations and services to negotiate which are locally based. It was agreed that localised information should be included in a thorough orientation. According to one participant, lack of orientation is:

> A major deficit in Queensland Health. A thorough orientation would make it very easy for the person that's coming in, to learn quickly. When I came there was no proper orientation, there were no rules about what I could and could not do although there was credentialing…but all it was, I just had to tick a few boxes and write one or two sentences explaining what I did and it was approved (Pascoe 2007).

One doctor felt that the role of a substantial, structured orientation program would ideally:

> Walk the IMG through every aspect of living and working in Australia like information about housing and schools to information on setting up a medical practice (Pascoe 2007).

How a medical practice is managed in Australia was particularly important for one participant who did not receive any related information during orientation:

> For me the main aspect is how you manage the practice itself. How you interact with patients, staff and community. What are the networks available? All these things need to be in your grasp before you even start the practice. Now you are put with someone for a couple of days and then you have to survive on your own (Pascoe 2007).

An additional comment was then made by a female participant: "We need all the information we can get so we can fight the system" (Pascoe 2007). I found this comment intriguing and wondered why the doctor felt she had to fight the system.

The final theme to emerge was that of working conditions. Aspects of working conditions such as supervision, work contracts and lack of access to Medicare were highlighted. The associated feelings were illustrated by participant experiences which encompassed vulnerability, powerlessness and the concept of cheap labour.

## Working Conditions

Medical practices are legally obliged to provide IMGs with supervision. Participants indicated that in their experience, many IMGs are left with very little or inappropriate supervision. When prompted to elaborate, one participant made the comment that: "Many of us feel like we've been thrown in at the deep end" (Pascoe 2007). All participating focus group members were critical of their supervision.

Another doctor added:

> The supervision given to me and to another IMG was mediocre to nothing and obviously the so called supervisor did not fit any guidelines. When this person did anything it was always criticism rather than assisting in finding out the problem and offering a solution. It happened because of the lack of guidelines and the lack of orientation (Pascoe 2007).

Another participant shared the experience of a colleague who had a personality clash with his supervisor. This eventually resulted in the IMG being dismissed from his duties. The IMG was not a permanent resident so was required to leave the country within 28 days because he was now without employment:

> The very next thing we had was people coming to our house crying, the whole family and they couldn't go back to where they'd come from, they'd sold everything from where they'd come from and what do they do, how do they get another job? (Pascoe 2007).

One participant raised work conditions embedded in contracts; this was of concern to all and discussed at length. Another IMG outlined his particular work situation:

> It is very prescriptive in the sense that IMGs have to do so many hours, see this many patients from this time to that time, and basically very little time is given to them for leave or to refresh themselves. I burn out. In our practice we work 8.30 to 5.30 every day and half day Saturday for the whole year with 6 weeks leave. I have worked for 4 years and I haven't had any leave. I can't there's no one there, no one running the place (Pascoe 2007).

One doctor commented that in some contracts, if leave is taken it is unpaid leave and often income received is based on the number of patients seen. It was pointed out that their colleagues employed by Queensland Health were paid for annual leave, while some IMGs employed by general practices were not. She stressed the importance of caring for self and family: "We must look at our quality of life, our partners, our families…take the leave if you need to do that" (Pascoe 2007). The IMG who had not taken any leave in 4 years replied:

It's easy to say but that's not the real thing because for a lot of people, they come here after leaving everything behind, they've sold everything and they want to restart and they want everything to be stabilised as quickly as possible and they need money for that. There is also a difference in where we come from and what we come to. There can be a big difference in our standard of living and those doctors who don't start as doctors, we find it more difficult (Pascoe 2007).

This prompted a participant to raise the vulnerability of IMGs particularly in relation to negotiating contracts:

You subconsciously say yes to most of the things that they want you to do rather than what you want. It is because of that vulnerable situation that we are put into and that's one thing we should address (Pascoe 2007).

Feeling powerless in the system was mentioned and the fact that many IMGs are reluctant to speak out. One doctor stated:

We come into a fragile situation that takes us out of our comfort zones, coming up from that takes a long time. Ideas spin in our minds, are we going to be deported because you make a wrong move? Have you missed your chance in life? Thus we are hesitant instead of saying this is what we want (Pascoe 2007).

The negotiation of a contract implies that both parties come to the table with equal bargaining powers. Many IMGs, however, feel vulnerable and some desperate to secure medical employment on any terms. Another participant believed that IMGs constitute a source of cheap labour:

The greatest percentage of bulk billing doctors are IMGs. People who want to start their practices as bulk billing, they look for IMGs because they are cheap labour. We are treated indirectly in a way as cheap labour. We are not cheaper labour; we have good skills, broad-based skills (Pascoe 2007).

The concept of cheap labour led to a short discussion on Medicare. While IMGs make a considerable contribution to healthcare services in the community, temporary resident IMGs cannot access Medicare benefits for themselves or their families. One doctor stated:

Most of us would be in the highest tax bracket and I find that very unfair. We contribute the most but don't get any benefit out of it (Pascoe 2007).

There have been many attempts over the years to secure Medicare benefits for temporary resident IMGs but to no avail; see (Haikerwal 2005). Another participant made the following analogy:

It's like having your own bakery but you cannot eat the bread in there (Pascoe 2007).

The focus group session concluded with some discussion about the Dr Patel case and the associated tragic events at the Bundaberg hospital. One participant believed that the Patel case has: "Put IMG/community relations back 20 years" (Pascoe 2007). It was felt that the Patel tragedy had undermined the general public's trust in IMGs. Another doctor stressed that:

Unfortunately, the general public sees an Indian doctor and tends to think we are all like him. This case has highlighted the deficiencies in Queensland Health rather than us (Pascoe 2007).

Final comments made reference to the need for more opportunities to meet with each other and to gather socially with families. It was mentioned that hospital doctors and doctors in general practice do not interact together. One doctor drew general agreement when he said: "New IMGs coming in should be introduced to the community, let's all get together" (Pascoe 2007). It seemed that the participating IMGs were feeling the need to connect with each other more often outside of professional/workplace contexts. There were a couple of opportunities for some humorous responses too (particularly some examples of their reactions to Australian slang). These experiences were advanced towards the end of our time together. Laughter was a nice informal way to conclude the session.

One doctor told of her confusion with the term 'runs' she said: "The patient said he has runs, I thought is he athlete? I had to ask the receptionist she said no it is diarrhoea!" (Pascoe 2007). Another doctor was concerned about his 'crook' patient: "He tells me he is crook…I don't want to know that you are a crook! I'm just here to provide you with medical treatment" (Pascoe 2007).

The focus group was instrumental in bringing together much of the observation, conversation and presentation I had been exposed to during my fieldwork at the ACRRM conference and the IMG forum. My next task was to undertake the individual interviews.

## The Interviews

The ten interviews I conducted were all unique experiences in terms of the settings and circumstances in which they occurred. Some participants came directly to Australia from their country of origin while others came via another country. I spoke with doctors who were rushing, doctors who were eating, doctors who were themselves unwell, doctors who did not want to share much information and doctors who could have talked for a much longer period.

The average age of participants was 41.7 years. One woman and two men participated in phone interviews, while the remainder of participants were interviewed face-to-face.

The following table introduces the interview cohort (Table 1):

I asked each participant for some demographic details and always began with the question prompt: *"Why did you come to Australia"?* This proved (as it did for the focus group) an effective way to get the conversation started. Barry's response (2011, interview 6) was one example:

In my country there was civil war, we had to leave for our kids for safety and English education, we came to beautiful Australia. They need me here too.

**Table 1**  Interview participants

| Participants (pseudonyms) | Sex | Age | Those who came via another country other than their own |
|---|---|---|---|
| Julian | M | 38 | |
| Colin | M | 41 | |
| Nancy | F | 47 | |
| Rita | F | 44 | Via New Zealand |
| Andrew | M | 41 | Via Canada |
| Barry | M | 40 | Via UK |
| Tania | F | 45 | Via South Africa |
| Shaun | M | 39 | |
| Gary | M | 35 | |
| Alex | M | 47 | Via New Zealand |

In the rest of the interview, I tried to keep as unstructured as possible, allowing the voice of the participant to direct the conversation. I wanted to create a space in which the doctor had freedom to voice what was most important for him or her. I also asked participants at the most appropriate time during the interview: *"Was there anything that shocked you about Australia?"* The most illuminating comment here was made by Julian who was visibly shocked when he shared the experience with me. On greeting him, one of Julian's first patients announced:

> Well finally someone from Europe, we're sick of those black ones from god knows where (2010, interview 1).

Being confronted with blatant racism on his first day at work was a shock. After repeating this testimony from a patient, Julian said: "This does not happen in Europe, I was just so shocked!"

Near the conclusion of the interview, I always asked the question: *"If a former colleague from your country contacted you about coming to work in Australia, what would you advise"?* I found that this question always provided an interesting range of responses. The responses were often quite lengthy and also included some humorous and surprising (from a Western perspective) advice. For example, Shaun wanted to alert his colleague to the terrible fact that: "They keep animals inside their houses here" (2012, interview 8). In Shaun's experience, having animals inside is out of the question and a serious health concern for humans.

I was surprised to learn that in Colin's country, driving a car is not necessarily the norm as it is in Australia. Colin, realising that driving is important in Australia, thought it is crucial for his colleague to: "Learn to drive before you come" (2010, interview 2).

Participants gave up what time they could or wanted to and revealed as much or as little of their experience as they wanted to. They shared their voices via the medium they selected. I was privileged to be invited into the personal spaces of the participants and privileged to be invited to hear their stories. I was also privileged to be able to view the stories of the doctors who made submissions to the Parliamentary Inquiry (2012) and Senate Committee (2016).

## The 2012 Parliamentary Inquiry—Lost in the Labyrinth

The motion for an inquiry was successfully put forward by Bruce Scott, member for Maranoa, on 18 October 2010. This occurred after much heated debate about various aspects related to the treatment of IMGs in Australia by the system. As a result, On Tuesday 23 November 2010, the then Minister for Health and Ageing, Hon. Nicola Roxon MP, announced that she would task the House of Representatives Standing Committee on Health and Ageing to inquire into and report on Registration Processes and Support for Overseas Trained Doctors.

The terms of reference for the Committee stated: "Recognising the vital role of colleges in setting and maintaining high standards for the registration of OTDs, the Committee will:

1. explore current administrative processes and accountability measures to determine if there are ways OTDs could better understand colleges' assessment processes, appeal mechanisms could be clarified, and the community better understand and accept registration decisions;
2. report on the support programs available through the Commonwealth and State and Territory governments, professional organisations and colleges to assist OTDs to meet registration requirements, and provide suggestions for the enhancement and integration of these programs; and
3. suggest ways to remove impediments and promote pathways for OTDs to achieve full Australian qualification, particularly in regional areas, without lowering the necessary standards required by colleges and regulatory bodies" (House of Representatives Standing Committee on Health and Ageing 2012).

The House of Representatives Standing Committee noted in its March 2012 Report entitled *Lost in the Labyrinth* the following significantly disturbing information: Almost one-third of IMGs who made submissions requested anonymity, citing fears that their chances of progressing through accreditation to registration would be compromised. The committee was also approached by IMGs, keen to share their views informally, but unable to make formal submissions fearing negative consequences (House of Representatives Standing Committee on Health and Ageing 2012, p. x).

The committee conducted 21 public hearings throughout Australia in every State and Territory in twelve different cities. The committee took direct evidence from 145 witnesses during the public hearings. They received 175 submissions from IMGs and interested others from across Australia as well as 22 supplementary submissions. From the total of 216 submissions, 109 were from IMGs and 91 from the various organisations and agencies involved in the registration, regulation, training and support of IMGs. The stories contributed additional, robust, data to the voices already at the centre of this study. I worked my way through the submissions with my primary focus on the 109 from IMGs. Although many of the submissions echoed aspects of experience which were also raised in the focus group and interviews of my study, these voices were different. IMGs recorded their experiences in writing to the inquiry committee. My interviews were largely unstructured, were less formal and included humour at times. In contrast, the experiences communicated in the submissions to the committee were first-hand accounts untouched or unfiltered by the influence of the researcher. Many were more focused on the journey or struggle with aspects of the system; they came directly from the IMG. Some submissions were stark accounts of disturbing experiences. I was in disbelief that medical practitioners in Australia could experience such unpleasant and even traumatic interactions and events that in the worse cases adversely impacted their physical and mental health.

Submissions made by other individuals, organisations and groups provided a rich source of background knowledge, opinions and critiques. These proved invaluable as I was able to gain an insight into how parts of the system viewed the current situation for IMGs as well as the recommendations they made to improve the registration processes for and support of these doctors. An additional source of data became available in 2016 by way of The Senate Community Affairs References Committee on Medical Complaints Process in Australia. On 2 February 2016, the Senate referred the medical complaints process to the committee for inquiry and report. The committee received 129 submissions and held two public hearings. Unlike the 2012 Parliamentary Inquiry which was tasked with inquiry related to IMGs specifically, this inquiry while receiving many submissions from IMGs was also open to submissions from Australian trained medical doctors, medical students, family members, organisations and associations. The 2016 Senate Inquiry's primary focus was on the intersection between bullying and harassment in Australia's medical profession and the medical complaints process. This timely inquiry was initiated at the same time as the voices in the media were revealing an ugly side of medicine, a toxic culture within the profession. The terms of reference for the committee below[4] show the broad scope of the inquiry: the prevalence of bullying and harassment in Australia's medical profession;

1. any barriers, whether real or perceived, to medical practitioners reporting bullying and harassment;
2. the roles of the Medical Board of Australia, the Australian Health Practitioners Regulation Agency and other relevant organisations in managing investigations into the professional conduct (including allegations of bullying and harassment), performance or health of a registered medical practitioner or student;
4. the operation of the *Health Practitioners Regulation National Law Act 2009* (the National Law), particularly as it relates to the complaints handling process;
5. whether the National Registration and Accreditation Scheme, established under the National Law, results in better health outcomes for patients and supports a world-class standard of medical care in Australia;

---

[4]https://www.aph.gov.au/Parliamentary_Business/Committees/Senate/Community_Affairs/Medical_Complaints/Terms_of_Reference.

6. the benefits of 'benchmarking' complaints about complication rates of particular medical practitioners against complication rates for the same procedure against other similarly qualified and experienced medical practitioners when assessing complaints;
7. the desirability of requiring complainants to sign a declaration that their complaint is being made in good faith; and
8. any related matters.

The submissions, along with the other data I collected, gave this study a broader and more comprehensive representation of the voice. Representation of voices in text, however, will always remain somewhat problematic. There is no perfect and exact representation as Lincoln and Denzin (1998, p. 407) reminded:

> At its heart lies an inner tension, an ongoing dialectic, a contradiction, that will never be resolved. On the one hand there is the concern for validity, or certainty in the text as a form of isomorphism and authenticity. On the other hand there is the sure and certain knowledge that all texts are socially, historically, politically, and culturally located. We, like the texts we write, can never be transcendent.

I was convinced to do the voices gifted to me justice, which I see as my responsibility; I needed a fresh approach. I viewed my responsibility as primarily to the participants in this study, not to a particular discipline or institution. As a result, I chose to adopt a multidisciplinary, social justice approach. A multidisciplinary approach was required to allow me to break free from the boundaries of one discipline. This in turn empowered me to give maximum representation to the voice; as much as the scope of a book will allow.

Following Foucault, Gariepy (2016) notes that if institutional and discipline politics result in the researcher reluctantly following established institutionalised paths, then the role of analysis tasked with uncovering relations of and vehicles for power is meaningless. The academy often reflects a biased view based on both quantitative and Eurocentric preferences. Rules and established standards are being applied to researcher conduct and research design in ways that are incompatible and hostile to non-quantitative approaches. For example, Brown and Strega (2005, p. 4) suggest that:

> By configuring research "subjects" in particular and limited ways, ethical review procedures are not only often problematic for social justice researchers but fail to consider ethical questions that are vitally important to them, such as voice, representation, and collaboration."

Ladson-Billings and Donnor (2005) join critical race theorists and others in the call for decolonisation of the academy, but question whether the academy has the ability to reconstruct itself into acceptance of a more flexible research framework. Foucault (1977, p. 207) made the following illuminating comment:

> Intellectuals are no longer needed by the masses to gain knowledge: the masses know perfectly well, without illusion; they know far better than the intellectual and they are certainly capable of expressing themselves. But there exists a system of power which blocks, prohibits, and invalidates this discourse and this knowledge, a power not only found in manifest authority of censorship, but one that profoundly and subtly penetrates an entire societal network.

> Intellectuals are themselves agents of this system of power-the idea of their responsibility for "consciousness" and discourse forms part of the system.

Feminist Patricia Hill Collins (1991, p. 261) advanced exactly the research qualities I was seeking: "personal accountability, caring, the value of individual expressiveness, the capacity for empathy and the sharing of emotionality". I was not looking to discover and advance truth; rather, I was seeking to uncover the knowledge constructed from IMG experience. I aligned myself with the intentions of Strega and Brown (2015, p. 6):

> Our intention is to contribute to the project of having research reflect, both in terms of its processes and in terms of the knowledge it constructs, the experience, expertise, and concerns of those who have traditionally been marginalised in the research process and by widely held beliefs about what "counts" as knowledge.

## Representation of the Voice

Brown and Strega (2005) (and Strega and Brown 2015) seek to situate social justice as mandatory for research processes and outcomes. Their appreciation of the political nature of research and push to understand different ways of being, knowing and doing resonate with me. Post-structuralism and feminist perspectives have contributed significantly to positionality, how the researcher positions themselves in relation to the participants in a study and reflexivity, the ongoing conversation the researcher has with themselves about interpretations of experiences. From a feminist post-structuralist stance, Brown and Strega (2005) critique the ontological and epistemological ideas of traditional social science and advance the potential of emancipatory research methodology.

This research does seek to privilege the IMG voice, the voice of the other. However, it must not silence, exclude, excuse or lose focus of the dominant power structures such as the system's role and influence in the construction of IMG experiences. The power differential became a central player in terms of exploring unequal social relations, systems and regimes. I agree with Choo and Ferree (2010, p. 136): "more attention to system-level complexity can enrich micro-level analysis, tightening the connections among power relations, institutional contexts and lived experience". Post-structuralism can be overly discourse-dependent in that explanation of the social order is reproduced in discourse as if discourse was the only vehicle. The notion of biopower explores the techniques of power and knowledge and their interrelationship. The effect of these relationships is manifested across conduct in public and political discourse (Gariepy 2016; Macias 2015, p. 232). The power of discourse should not be underestimated but not so clear is: "...how, why and by what social forces do some discourses supersede others and become hegemonic and thus organising and ruling documents" (Aguiar 2012, p. 16). Ongoing patterns of economic inequalities between groups, for example, are not only situated within the economy via discourse but also in unequal access to the valued goods of society. Intersectionality offered an emancipatory, anti-oppressive framework for the exploration of intersecting social phenomena and was therefore the best way to organise and explain the experiences of IMGs in Australia. Participants in this study raised several critical issues which must not only impact on their integration into and retention in rural and remote practice, but also on the very well-being of the doctors and their families. This data set builds into themes and key ideas for discussion and exploration in subsequent chapters. This chapter has outlined the emergent design of the study. The participants have been introduced to the reader and my role and perspective as researcher has been discussed. The process of data collection and important ethical considerations has also been raised.

# References

Absolon, K., & Willett, C. (2005). Putting ourselves forward: Location in aboriginal research. In L. Brown & S. Strega (Eds.), *Research as resistance: Critical, indigenous, and anti-oppressive approaches* (pp. 97–126). Canadian scholars' press, Toronto.

Aguiar, L. L. M. (2012). Redirecting the academic gaze upward. In L. L. M. Aguiar & C. J. Schneider (Eds.), *Researching amongst elites: Challenges and opportunities in studying up* (pp. 1–27). UK: Ashgate publishing.

Australian Rural and Remote Workforce Agencies Group. (2005). *Submission to the productivity commission on health workforce* (pp. 1–39). Viewed 15 June 2011. http://www.pc.gov.au/inquir ies/completed/health-workforce/submissions/sub136/136.pdf.

Berg, B. (2004). *Qualitative research methods for the social sciences* (5th ed.). Boston: Pearson education.

Brown, L., & Strega, S. (2005). *Research as resistance: Critical, indigenous and anti-oppressive approaches*. Toronto: Canadian Scholars' Press.

Choo, H. Y., & Ferree, M. M. (2010). Practicing intersectionality in sociological research. *Sociological Theory, 28*(2), 129–149.

Crenshaw, K. (1991). Mapping the margins: Intersectionality, identity politics, and violence against women of color. *Stanford Law Review, 43*, 1241–1299.

Foucault, M. (1977). *Language, counter-memory, practice*. Ithaca, NY: Cornell University Press.

Gariepy, K. D. (2016). *Power, discourse, ethics: A policy study of academic freedom*. Sense Publishers, Rotterdam, The Netherlands. Viewed 5 May 2017. https://www.sensepublishers.com.

Gilding, M. (2010). Motives of the rich and powerful in doing interviews with social scientists. *International Sociology, 25*(6), 755–77. Viewed October 12, 2015, https://doi.org/10.1177/0268 580909351323, http://iss.sagepub.com/content/25/6/755.

Haikerwal, M. (2005). *Observations from an overseas trained doctor*. Australian Medical Association. Viewed 5 April 2007. http://www.ama.com.au/web.nsf/doc/WEEN-6EG7CN.

Hawthorne, L., Birrell, B., & Young, D. (2004). The retention of overseas trained doctors in general practice in regional Victoria, pp. 1–100.

Hertz, R., & Imber, J. B. (1993). Fieldwork in elite settings (introduction). *Journal of Contemporary Ethnography, 22*(1), 3–6.

Hill Collins, P. (1991). *Black feminist thought: Knowledge, consciousness, and the politics of empowerment*. Boston, MA: Unwin Hyman.

Hill Collins, P. (2013). *On intellectual activism*. Philadelphia: Temple University Press.

Hiller, H. H. (1996). *Canadian society: A macro analysis*. Scarborough, ON: Prentice Hall.

House of Representatives Standing Committee on Health and Ageing. (2012). *Lost in the Labyrinth: Report on the inquiry into registration processes and support for overseas trained doctors*. The Parliament of the Commonwealth of Australia, Canberra.

Kamberelis, G., & Dimitriadis, G. (2008). Focus groups: Strategic articulations of pedagogy, politics and inquiry. In N. K. Denzin & Y. S. Lincoln (Eds.), *Collecting and interpreting qualitataive materials* (3rd ed., pp. 375–402). Thousand Oaks, CA: Sage Publications.

Kaomea, J. (2004). Dilemmas of an indigenous academic: A native Hawaiian story. In K. Mutua & B. B. Swadener (Eds.), *Decolonizing research in cross-cultural contexts: Critical personal narratives* (pp. 27–44). Albany: State University of New York Press.

Knowles, R. (2015). *Expert advisory group draft report on discrimination, bullying and sexual harassment.* Melbourne: Royal Australasian College of Surgeons. https://www.surgeons.org/me dia/22045685eag-report-to-racs-draft-08-sept-2015.pdf.

Krueger, R. A. (1994). *Focus groups: A practical guide for applied research* (2nd ed.). Thousand Oaks, CA: Sage Publications.

Ladson-Billings, G. (2003). Racialized discourses and ethnic epistemologies. In N. K. Denzin & Y. S. Lincoln (Eds.), *The landscape of qualitative research: Theories and issues* (2nd ed., pp. 398–432). Thousand Oaks, CA: Sage Publications.

Ladson-Billings, G., & Donnor, J. (2005). The moral activist role of critical race theory scholarship. In N. K. Denzin & Y. S. Lincoln (Eds.), *Sage handbook of qualitative research* (3rd ed., pp. 279–302). Thousand Oaks, CA: Sage.

Lincoln, Y. S., & Denzin, N. K. (1998). The fifth moment. In N. K. Denzin & Y. S. Lincoln (Eds.), *The landscape of qualitative research: Theories and issues* (pp. 407–429). Thousand Oaks: Sage Publications.

Macias, T. (2015). On the Footsteps of Foucault: Doing foucauldian discourse analysis in social justice research. In S. Strega & L. Brown (Eds.), *Research as resistance: Revisiting critical, indigenous, and anti-oppressive approaches* (2nd ed., pp. 221–242). Toronto: Canadian Scholars' Press.

Magnat, V. (2012). Productive disorientation, or the ups and downs of embodied research. In L. L. M. Aguiar & C. J. Schneider (Eds.), *Researching amongst elites: Challenges and opportunities in studying up* (pp. 179–197). Surrey: Ashgate publishing.

Mills, C. W. (1956). *The power elite.* New York: Oxford University Press.

Ortner, S. (2010). Access: Reflections on studying up in hollywood. *Ethnography, 11*(2), 211–233.

Pakulski, J. (2011). Global elites. In J.A. Agnew & J.S. Duncan (Eds), *The wiley-blackwell companion to human geography* (pp. 328–45). Malden, MA: Blackwell.

Pascoe, V.A. (2007). *International medical graduates—Focus group.* X Division of General Practice.

Pascoe, V.A. (2011). *Experiences of culture shock, vulnerability and powerlessness: Reflections from international medical graduates and the impact on their wellbeing.* Paper presented to 2011 Migration Update South Australia and Beyond, Adelaide, 23–24 June 2011.

Roffee, J.A. (2016). Rhetoric, Aboriginal Australians and the Northern Territory intervention: A socio-legal investigation into pre-legislative argumentation. *International Journal for Crime, Justice and Social Democracy.* Viewed 22 April 2017, http://www.healthinfonet.ecu.edu.au/upl oads/resources/3113-3113.pdf.

Savage, M., & Williams, K. (2008). Elites remembered in capitalism and forgotten by social sciences. In M. Savage & K. Williams (Eds.), *Remembering elites* (pp. 1–24). Malden, MA: Blackwell.

Smith, L. T. (1999). *Decolonizing methodologies: Research and indigenous peoples.* London: Zed Books.

Stake, R. E. (2000). Case studies. In N. K. Denzin & Y. S. Lincoln (Eds.), *Handbook of qualitative research* (2nd ed., pp. 435–454). Thousand Oaks, CA: Sage Publications.

Strega, S. (2015). The view from the poststructural margins: Epistemology and methodology reconsidered. In S. Strega & L. Brown (Eds.), *Research as resistance, revisiting critical, indigenous, and anti-oppressive approaches* (2nd ed., pp. 119–152). Toronto: Canadian Scholars' Press.

Strega, S., & Brown, L. (Eds.). (2015). *Research as resistance: Revisiting critical, indigenous, and anti-oppressive approaches.* Toronto: Canadian Scholar's Press.

The Senate Community Affairs References Committee. (2016). *Medical complaints process in Australia,* Canberra. https://www.ap.gov.au/Parliamentary_Business/Committees/Senate/Comm unity_Affairs/MedicalComplaints45.

Tomic, P., & Trumper, R. (2012). Methodological challenges faced when researching in hostile environments: The SAWP in a Canadian Hinterland. In L. L. M. Aguiar & C. J. Schneider (Eds.), *Researching amongst elites: Challenges and opportunities in studying up* (pp. 233–252). Surrey: Ashgate Publishing.

Vagle, M. D. (2014). *Crafting phenomenological research*. Walnut Creek, CA: Left coast press inc.

Vidich, A. J., & Lyman, S. M. (2003). Qualitative methods: Their history in sociology and anthropology. In N. K. Denzin & Y. S. Lincoln (Eds.), *The landscape of qualitative research: Theories and issues* (2nd ed., pp. 55–129). Thousand Oaks, CA: Sage Publications.

Willis, E., Reynolds, L., & Keleher, H. (Eds.). (2016). *Understanding the Australian health care system* (3rd ed.). Chatswood, NSW: Elsevier.

# The Lucky Country: IMGs and the History of Ethnocentrism, Xenophobia and Racism

Australia was invaded at the time of the heyday of unrestricted medical practice in Britain...unfettered by government intervention. Doctors in this period did not enjoy particularly high social status. British healers were a diverse lot... the physician, the surgeon, the barber, the bonesetter, the empiric, the midwife and the apothecary (Martyr 2002, p. 191).

After two hundred years of medicine in Australia, no effort is spared to impose uniformity on the selection of those who would aspire to study medicine; and the training and standards of today's Medical Schools lead to a great uniformity not only in technical skills, but in professional outlook and style (Pearn 1988, p.33).

## Introduction

Historical analysis can make a fundamental contribution towards understanding the present. Sociologists such as founding father Auguste Comte and later contemporary thinker C. Wright Mills particularly stressed the importance of both history and biography. Karl Marx (and Comte) believed that history was created in stages, with each stage consisting of the seeds for the next. Therefore, initially, a background history is provided to set the scene and flag significant stages. An appreciation of how Australia has evolved through the exploration of important influences and events that have helped shape the Australian nation provides the reader with a context for discussion. This chapter outlines the journey of Western medicine in Australia from the discovery of the Great Southern Land and the medical practices of Indigenous Australians, to the arrival of the first IMGs, the arrival of refugee IMGs, to the current context of medical practice. Themes of class, race and nation assist to reveal the foundations of theme development and their intersection in the positioning of IMGs in medical practice and within Australian society. The emergence of the medical profession as a high-status, powerful force with the ability to successfully lobby governments to further its own agenda becomes evident. The position of status and power afforded to Australian trained medical doctors is perpetuated

© Springer Nature Singapore Pte Ltd. 2019
V. A. Pascoe, *Australia's Toxic Medical Culture*,
https://doi.org/10.1007/978-981-13-2426-0_3

and reinforced via the development of the Australian nation and associated racism, xenophobia and ethnocentrism. History shows the development of a fearful nation, one which feels threatened by 'others'. Subsequently, medical doctors trained overseas began to be regarded with suspicion, eventually resulting in the perception of an inferior underclass status where their training and qualifications are questionable. This chapter reveals the emergence of an entrenched pattern of well-documented, deliberate, long-standing discrimination against IMGs.

## In the Beginning: The Invasion of an Ancient Land

It was the Dutchman Willem Janszoon of the Dutch East India Company who sighted the Western Australian coast in 1606. Decades later in 1688 the first Englishman, William Dampier, set foot on the continent (Blong et al. 2016). Modern European exploration built to a climax in the nineteenth century. Etherington and MacKenzie (2016, p. 1) state that: "By this time exploration was ideologically charged, closely bound up with the extension of western empires, of white settlement across the world, as well as the development of all forms of scientific study". Dampier observed Indigenous Australians and described them as: "The miserablest people in the world, thus starting a trend to place them on the lowest rung of the scale of humanity" (Muecke and Shoemaker 2004, p. 13). Englishman Captain James Cook was instructed to continue to search for the Great Southern Land. On 21 August 1770, he landed on the east coast and in the name of King George the third took 'possession' (Steinberg 2016). It was not until January 1788, however, that the first fleet arrived in Australia at Botany Bay. The Australian continent represented a new solution for convict transportation and became a penal colony. The first fleet numbered 1350 people, 759 of those were convicts. The voyage from England covered 15,000 miles and took 8 months and 1 week. There were forty-eight deaths including seventeen convicts who died before the fleet left England (Nugent 2003; Simpson 1988). Quigley (2017, p. 139) notes: "approximately one hundred and sixty thousand convicts were transported from the British Isles to Australia in the period 1787–1868". The new boat arrivals found a vast and diverse country with a challenging climate. The convicts who arrived in Australia were from the 'causal poor' and most were hardened criminals due to the harsh conditions they experienced in England. The new society they now found themselves in was an authoritarian society that further brutalised them, and there was a deep divide between the free and the penal. Broom (1994, p. 24) explains:

> They were generally seen as inferior and useless by the gaolers and used as cheap labour. About 40 per cent of all male convicts in Australia were flogged for some misdemeanour...- Less than one in five of the convicts were women, and even they were generally made as callous as the men by the environment that produced them.

From these very new beginnings in a 'new' land, class division and discrimination with associated perceptions of who constituted superior and inferior peoples was quickly established, but what of the existing population, Australia's Indigenous population? The Great Southern Land was also an ancient land (Breen 2008). Australia was the last continent discovered by Europeans but was the first continent for the Indigenous inhabitants.

## Australia's First Peoples

Indigenous Australians were the first peoples to occupy this country and their habitation of the Australian continent constitutes the longest continual occupation by an ancient culture anywhere on earth (Muecke and Shoemaker 2004). Evidence gained through the use of radiocarbon dating on artefacts and human remains confirmed Indigenous occupation of Australia for at least 60,000 years. How much earlier according to Broom (1994) is unclear but charcoal dated at 100,000 years was found near Lake George in Canberra, possibly confirmation of human habitation. Moreover, Maxwell-Stewart (2016, p. 359) claims that Australia's "geological history extends a further 3070 million years".

Many Indigenous people, however, reject this Western view and believe that Indigenous Australians were created by the ancestral spirit beings. These supernatural beings also created the earth and the flora and fauna during the Dreamtime, which occurred at the beginning of time (Arbon 2008; Devere et al. 2017). The beginning of time does not have a date, and many Indigenous people dispute the established Western ideas around migration theories (Stanner 1987). For example, many historians believe that Indigenous people arrived in Australia during the Pleistocene period when low sea levels allowed access from Southeast Asia via the Indonesian Archipelago. Many Indigenous people do not acknowledge a heritage that has origins outside of Australia. "Their heritage is of being here as if forever" (Partington 1998, p. 27). Country for an Indigenous Australian was a complex idea. Dunn (2017, p. 76) explains the concept of country as:

> An interweaving of physical, territorial and cultural understandings of a place. While it could indeed refer to the physical landscape, country was more multidimensional as it also identified the people who lived in or managed an area, the animals, the waterways, the earth, the soil, the sky and the underground. Everyone had a country, an area of land defined by their sites and knowledge and under the care and management of a particular group. In their own country, a person might see the landscape shaped through their understanding of the Dreaming and filled with sites and stories that explained the logic of the place.

When Europeans invaded in 1788, there were approximately 300,000 Indigenous Australians living in Australia. The population was divided into over 500 tribes each with their own distinct territory, history, dialect, customs and culture (Broom 1994, p. 11). Therefore, it can be argued that multiculturalism is not a relatively new concept in Australia. Indigenous societies and their structures show that the continent has always been divided into many different, distinct Indigenous nations (Shellam et al. 2017). Moreover, Indigenous Australians view and identify with Australia and each other in relation to this perspective which still exists strongly today (see the map of Aboriginal Australia, Horton 1996).

At the time of invasion, Indigenous populations were highly concentrated in coastal areas where there was an abundance of food resources, water and shelter. In desert areas, other Indigenous populations managed to adapt to the conditions. "Over millennia the first Australians succeeded to develop strategies for a nomadic, hunter-gatherer lifestyle whether they were located in rainforests, on coastal fore-shores, in cold alpine regions or in arid seemingly waterless deserts" (Covacevich 1990, p. 61). Indigenous Australians had contact with close neighbours from the north such as Torres Strait Islander peoples and peoples from Papua New Guinea and the Indonesian islands. The first Australians also established trade relationships with their neighbours. For example, Macassan fisherman negotiated with the peoples of Arnhem Land to harvest trepang[1] in Australia's north. The seasonal visits from these neighbours also provided trade and skill exchange opportunities (Shellam et al. 2017). European invaders changed the country and the way of life of the traditional owners; they became the dominant power. Australia's first peoples and the invaders were culturally poles apart.

Indigenous Australians had survived for thousands of years in a non-materialist ethos which embraced continuity over change, whereas the European invaders came with a background of divide and conquer and the entrenched ideals of change and development conducive to an industrial society. Indigenous cultures were under-mined by the frontier of intrusion perpetuated by the invaders who brought about the massacre and dispossession from land of many Indigenous peoples throughout Australia (Broom 1994; Lippmann 1991; Nettelback 2017; Reynolds 1987, 2013). As a result, culture and language were lost on a genocidal level (Partington 1998). According to Lippmann (1991), the Europeans did not place any value on Indigenous cultures. Indigenous peoples were described by the invaders as: "wandering bands of savages still living in the Stone Age. This perception was the beginning of a deep and long-lasting cultural misapprehension" (Muecke and Shoemaker 2004, p. 11). The invaders had no idea that they were disrupting highly structured knowledge systems, as Sykes (1986, p. 30) explained:

> In traditional society, there were many highly skilled people – not only doctors and lawyers, but teachers, geographers, chemists, botanists, and people trained in communications (not only with the living, but also with nature and the spirit world). We had linguists, historians, etc., and while everybody was obliged to learn a little about most of these things, it was the lifetime duty of some people to carry the whole knowledge of each subject and pass it on to whoever would be replacing them.

Doctors or healers in Indigenous Australian cultures were the only authentic, legitimate medical practitioners in the ancient Australian continent until Europeans arrived (Reid et al. 2016). Their ancient healing practices existed well before the development of Western medicine: "Contemporary oral history of surviving Abo-riginal lore provides a glimpse of the world's longest surviving medical practices ... these medical procedures predate the teachings of Hippocrates and Galen, not by

---

[1] A seafood delicacy also known as beche-de-mer or sea cucumber.

centuries but by millennia"[2] (Covacevich 1990, p. 61). The Indigenous healer held great power and was awarded great respect. Indigenous Australians today may still seek treatment from traditional healers. As Reid et al. (2016, p. 154) note:

> While Indigenous healers might now be contacted by phone, the principles underlying their practice remain consistent and tied to the unique but diverse world-views of Indigenous peoples. Indigenous or traditional healers are generally identified by other healers and then educated in the practice, which focuses largely on maintaining holistic well-being. Physical, psychological and social well-being are integrated in Indigenous conceptualisations of health, and this traditional model still operates today throughout some parts of Australia.

Some Europeans embraced aspects of Indigenous healing especially herbal/plant remedies which, because they had been developed for the Australian context, were more effective. Others, however, dismissed it as "witchcraft and mumbo-jumbo … yet this medicine like other forms of non-orthodox health care has still survived" (Martyr 2002, p. 15). Over time, traditional medicine was systematically overwhelmed but not eliminated by the new Western medical regime. The first medical doctors trained overseas to come to Australia were naval surgeons and explorers.

## The First IMGs

Naval surgeons accompanied the exploration expeditions that mapped the Australian coast. Upon arrival in 1788, the first fleet had a company of nine doctors. Surgeon John Irving came with the first fleet as a convict (convicted for grand larceny) and served as the surgeon on the Prince of Wales; he eventually became the first convict in New South Wales to be emancipated (Simpson 1988). Not all surgeons did as well as John Irving; while some came with good surgical backgrounds, others came with questionable surgical backgrounds and unstable personalities. Some did not arrive at all, such as the inebriated surgeon who cut his own throat five days after his ship The Clifton set sail from England (Woolcock 1988). Others fell into disrepute after arrival in Australia such as Irish surgeon James Murray who became a psychopath and, murderer and as a result, was rejected as a member of the medical profession. Some surgeons went on to occupy different roles such as Jamison, Balmain and Arndell who all became magistrates. Some surgeons became philanthropists and wealthy landowners. Scottish surgeon Daniel Curdie became a Senator of Melbourne University, and Englishman George Bennett was a founder of the Faculty of Medicine at the University of Sydney (Pearn 1988; Pearn and Cobcroft 1990). Due to the penal nature of the colony, for 50 years after 1788: "The crown supplied almost all medical care for free settlers, as well as convicts, through the salaried Colonial Medical Service (CMS)" (Lewis 2014, p. S5). In her discussion of the history of

---

[2]Greek physician Hippocrates (600–500 BC) developed the forerunner of Western medicine based on reason rather than religion. Galen (130–200 AD) furthered Hippocratic beliefs and established a medical tradition that lasted for the next 1000 years by merging all existing medical knowledge at the time.

medicine in Australia, Martyr (2002, p. 26) claims: "Immigrants, convicts and ship's doctors … brought with them all the hotch-potch conventional wisdoms, empiricism, rationalism, pseudo-science and inspired guesswork that made up British medicine in the late 1700s".

The ship's surgeon was required to treat all those on-board ships, from convicts to vice-regal patients (Pearn 1988). The most common diseases suffered by passengers were transmitted by infected arthropod species such as mosquitoes, fleas and ticks and consisted of infections or parasitic illnesses. Venereal diseases were also common as well as pulmonary diseases such as tuberculosis and nutritional diseases such as scurvy (Cossart 2014; Mcleod 1988). Medical treatment at the time would, by today's standards, be considered barbaric and included clinical methods such as bloodletting, restraining, blistering and purging. Women were also the carers at home, where they nursed the sick, made up home remedies, delivered babies and were agents in disease prevention (Doherty 2016). They provided the primary care in the early days of the colony, and there were self-help medical books available to inform diagnosis and treatment such as The Poor Man's Medicine Chest (1791). The contribution of women to healing went mostly unrecorded (Martyr 2002). As the colony grew, there were not enough doctors. Many people learned to either do without medical advice or accessed untrained and non-registered health practitioners, as the distance to travel to see a trained doctor could take as long as one week.

Scientific enquiry further developed which in turn expanded medical knowledge of disease and treatments (Cossart 2014; Thearle 1990). According to Lawrence and Brown (2016, p. 150):

> Ideas of scientific exploration were fuelling a generation of men who opened the world to colonization and when surgeons were beginning to establish themselves as the major social and therapeutic presence in urban medicine.

Formal medical qualifications as required by today's standards, however, did not exist in 1788. In fact, it was not until the Medical Act of 1858 that English and Scottish doctors received university-based training. Instead, medical students received most of their training through apprenticeship to a practitioner. "Many who completed their articles of apprenticeship went to medical school to 'top up' their medical training but many were not awarded a formal degree in medicine" (Pearn and Cobcroft 1990, p. 51). As Lewis (2014, p. S5) notes:

> Under the early colonial economic and social conditions, the traditional English division of the profession into status groups of physicians, surgeons and apothecaries (recognised from 1815 in England as general practitioners) could simply not be transplanted.

It was not until the end of the nineteenth century, however, that the foundation of medicine as practised in today's society was laid (Lawrence and Brown 2016; Thearle 1990). After the colony was established, one of the primary tasks for Governor Phillip (governor from 1788–1792) was to explore and map the continent. Exploration parties were accompanied by a doctor. Unlike the naval surgeons, these doctors were civilians who sought adventure. Pearn and Cobcroft (1990, p. 59) note that: "Medicine has always been a passport to adventure and to a wider world". The doctor explorers had an interest in natural history and the discovery of new plants and animals. Some were also interested in Indigenous Australians and several of them recorded languages. In some instances, these records were of languages now lost (Pearn and Cobcroft 1990). There was much about the unique Australian environment to learn however and in terms of medicine, especially preventive medicine; the newcomers remained virtually ignorant of the already established practices of Australia's Indigenous peoples.

> The lifestyles and medical practices of the Australian Aborigines had solved many of the problems which were to reappear when new waves of immigrants…pushed into the unknown in the 19th century. Many of the lessons of preventive medicine, formally evolved over millennia, had to be relearned by the often paternalistic and patronising…who displaced the original inhabitants (Pearn and Cobcroft 1990, p. iv).

Many convicts arrived already diseased (Cossart 2014; Lewis 2014). Common illnesses thrived such as diarrhoea and scurvy (Quigley 2017). As described by Charles Bowly: "My hands are hardly ever sound; the sun burns them into sores and then the place festers and spreads gradually over the back of the hand…it is produced from a want of fresh vegetables" (Martyr 2002, p. 35). Indigenous Australians did not suffer from scurvy while they were able to continue a hunter–gather lifestyle based on intimate knowledge of local food sources. Unfortunately though, Indigenous Australians did not possess any immunity to the new diseases and when traditional food quest practices were also impacted there were many deaths. Broom (1994, p. 58) explains:

> Once contact was made with Europeans…smallpox, influenza, measles and the common cold swept away many Aborigines. Even 20 years after first contact epidemics raged…lung and chest complaints killed hundreds…and later tuberculosis…and the most insidious infection venereal disease. Static living and their new diet not only caused malnutrition, but appeared to raise their blood pressure, cholesterol levels and induce diabetes.

There was much illness and disease for the new IMGs to treat but the colony depended upon imported drugs which could: "melt, become rancid or otherwise decompose en route, making them unreliable, and adding to the unpredictability of medical treatment" (Martyr 2002, p. 39). The new environment must have been extremely challenging in terms of not only medical practice but also the stark change in climate, lifestyle and geographic isolation. How did IMGs adjust, did they find a solidarity among themselves? Did they have power and high status in the new colony?

## Class

Lawrence and Brown (2016, pp. 149–150) in their discussion of the centralising role of the professions and science in colonisation argue that: "Surgeons boasted that their profession offered the opportunity for ordinary men to rise in society. Along with geographical explorers, they pointed to the modest origin of many of their number". Some Australian and British historians hold the view that doctors who went to the colonies were second rate and as a result could not find work in Britain. Doctors debarred in the UK were allowed to practise in the colonies without penalty. In British medical culture at the time, one could be an excellent doctor but if one did not have the essential connections within the profession, the opportunity to emigrate could become an attractive option. Martyr (2002, p. 42) argues:

> British medical culture in the 1800 s was exclusive, and best served by those who had an entrée to the right medical schools, hospitals and societies. A hint toward this can be found in often anti-establishment views expressed in Australian medical journalism of the 19th century, where the insular and elitist nature of the British medical world is frequently criticised.

This implies that the first IMGs became a cohesive professional group. Perhaps the vast distance between England and Australia also allowed IMGs to distance themselves from their past colleagues and the established British medical culture. Perhaps an IMG without the essential connections in British medical terms could be empowered in the new colony? It can be argued that despite their diversity, the first fleet surgeons did find a sense of professional solidarity. Archives provide evidence of this when surgeon Arthur Bowes Smyth on 11 February 1788 recorded the search for local plants to treat scurvy. His writing referred to colleagues as: "the Gentlemen of the Faculty in the Settlement". This indicated that the first fleet surgeons regarded themselves as a 'Faculty' as in the 'Faculty of Medicine' (Pearn 1988, p. 53). Lewis (2014, p. S6) argues that "colonial doctors were eager to establish external symbols of solidarity, as well as to defend themselves against the considerable competition from irregulars". This was an imperative as the public was able to choose between orthodox and unorthodox practitioners.

Despite surgeons being considered as men of the Settlement Upper Class, some married convicts (Pearn 1988). For example, Thomas Arndell married his convict housekeeper and mother of their six children in 1807. Even the most senior surgeon, General John White married a convict. Acceptance by a professional upper class for marriage with convicts was previously unheard of. Pearn (1988, p. 54) argues: "marriage with convicts, by their personal example, cannot be overstated as one of the significant socialising influences operative in that society". However, while some surgeons lived comfortable lives with convict partners, some did not provide for their widows to care for their families after they had died. Perhaps some of these marriages did not attract the level of commitment and responsibility usually associated with a 'good' marriage made in England.

The new arrivals were born, raised and socialised into the highly structured class system of their homelands, and some of these traditions and prejudices were bound to transfer to the colonies. They were fiercely divided by ethnicity and religion and were known as belonging to the three kingdoms (English, Scots and Irish). Hirst (2014, p. 143) asserts that: "In their home countries they had long been enemies of one another". In addition, they were divided between Catholic and Protestant. The new immigrants provided their labour power to build a new nation aligned with a capitalist system. "The new nation had a class structure and race, cultural and gender relations that reflected the dominant groups and their interests, and the society was stratified in terms of race, ethnicity, gender and class" (Pettman 1992, p. 7). Science and medicine and associated developments supported the emerging structure of the new Australian nation.

Fashions in science and medicine assisted the justification and perpetuation of old entrenched ideas. Phrenology, developed by German physician Franz Gall, is a good example. This science was used in early nineteenth century Australian penal and medical practice. Phrenology sought to prove that the size and form of the skull were related to the brain and personality. The measuring of skulls, especially so-called primitive skulls, became an obsession with phrenologists who claimed that level of intelligence, the cause of insanity and the predisposition to commit crimes were all related to brain size (Hughes 2017; Van Wyhe 2004). Phrenology had significant influence in the formation of opinion and was used to justify the idea of European superiority over so-called lesser races such as the Maori of New Zealand and Australia's Indigenous population, which were classified as physiologically criminal (Broom 1994). Phrenology also served to uphold old prejudices as Martyr (2002, p. 51) argues: "To spot a criminal type also simply confirmed existing prejudices of racial inferiority and inherent criminality, not just of non-whites but of the Irish and Welch". Phrenology was discredited by 1848, and Martyr (2002, p. 48) states that it constituted: "a profound embarrassment in the history of science and the history of medicine". Charles Darwin's Origin of Species (1859) when manipulated to suit the inferiority agenda also constituted a convenient theory to absolve European Australians from responsibility for the decline of the Indigenous population. Darwin proposed survival of the fittest to explain evolution in the plant and animal worlds. Many who claimed superiority of the white race argued that Darwin's ideas offered an explanation for the depopulation of black races as a result of the process of European colonisation (see Van Wyhe 2004). The expansion of this myth led to some bizarre claims, even from reportedly reputable sources such as the Australasian Anthropological Journal which in 1896 alleged:

> Once Aborigines passed puberty 'the sutures of the cranium begin to consolidate, and the forepart of the brain ceases to develop as it does in other races'. By the end of the nineteenth century, the general public became very familiar with phrases like 'survival of the fittest' and 'white superiority'. That was all the theory they needed to support their simple and popular form of racist thinking (Broom 1994, p. 93).

The first Australians found themselves reduced to an ethnic minority in their own country; they were relegated to an underclass position which persisted over time and still remains today. Narratives of 'Australianness' often omit Indigenous histories and identities from nationalist discourse. Plage et al. (2016, p. 3) in their discussion on cosmopolitanism, nationalism and the concept of a 'fair go' state: "Eurocentric or neo-colonial cosmopolitanism may normalize previous colonial relationships at the expense of Indigenous populations". In fact, Indigenous Australians were virtually dismissed by the dominant society and were not even officially counted in the census until 1967 (Gunstone 2017; Pettman 1992). A large wave of Chinese attracted to the goldfields during the 1850s saw the arrival of a new ethnic minority which was quickly assigned an inferior status and relegated to another underclass (Beattie 2016). Walker

(1999, p. 2) argues that: "the Chinese were commonly depicted as the forerunners of a subtle invasion". Moreover, Australia has always managed to racialise different groups at different times. Following a 1991 Human Rights and Equal Opportunity Commission report, Pettman (1992, p. 9) sums up:

> In Australia in the late nineteenth century not only the Chinese but also the Irish were represented as belonging to a race apart, presumed to have essential qualities by virtue of their birth identities. In the 1930 s Italians were not white enough; and post-Second World War migrants from southern Europe were also singled out, though more often using language or country of origin to predict otherness. 'Asians' became the most visible non-Aboriginal targets of racism in the 1980 s, while Muslim and Arab Australians are the most recent groups to be racialized and victimised.

I argue that IMGs, too, became an underclass and came to be viewed as such within the medical profession in Australia. As the new dominant society in the colony evolved and developed, the first IMGs became the established Australian medical profession. After the emergence of the first Australian medical school at the University of Melbourne in 1862 (Lewis 2014), the profession in Australia, built on the foundations of the first IMGs, now graduated the first Australian trained doctors. As the colony became more westernised, the IMGs who now arrived from overseas became labelled as foreign. Subsequently, the long history of IMGs as an underclass within an elite profession began. This was particularly prevalent during periods of war and the subsequent immigration of displaced persons. As a result, many doctors now arrived in Australia as refugees.

## Refugee IMGs

During the First World War (1914–1918), people of German origin in Australia, including doctors trained in Germany and practising in Australia, bore the brunt of anti-German sentiment. A xenophobic mindset developed and consequently a non-acceptance of doctors now considered medical outsiders. Kamien (2006) believes that this was especially evident if IMGs threatened the 'medical turf' of Australian trained doctors. In the 1930s, due to the persecution of Jewish populations in Europe, Australia experienced a cohort of fleeing refugee Jewish doctors from Germany as well as countries such as Russia, Poland and Austria (Iredale 2009). The Second World War (1939–1945) created a catastrophic dislocation of populations in Europe with an unprecedented 12 million people made homeless (Kunz 1975; Markus and Semyonov 2010). Many people in Europe, while not seeking refuge from ethnic persecution, sought refuge from new adverse political change (Glynn and Kleist 2012). Post-war Australia was in desperate need to boost the labour force and felt particularly vulnerable (especially from the 'yellow peril' of the pacific) as a large country with a small population of approximately seven million (Hirst 2014, p. 152). The realisation of Australia's close proximity to Asia was especially heightened by the Japanese advances on the Australian coast during the war. Walker (1999, pp 3–4) sums up views at the time:

> Australia appeared as a vulnerable continent subject either to direct attack from the East or
> to a more gradual loss of its British heritage at the hands of Asian intruders…Australians
> saw themselves as an outpost of Europe facing Asia.

These circumstances led the Australian Government to introduce a displaced persons migration scheme (Maley 2016; Panayi 2016). Determined to, as rapidly as possible, increase the Australian population, the scheme was fully government sponsored. According to Kunz (1975, p. 1), "Australia admitted 170,000 Displaced Persons, one of the most prominent countries of resettlement, running second only to the United States". This resulted in an influx of displaced persons which exposed Australians, who had mostly taken on British norms and values, to a tide of diverse non-British outsiders. Kunz (1975, p. 2) contends that: "displaced persons became human guinea pigs on whom was tested the social and political feasibility of the government's intention". This was a new and challenging situation for Australia; displaced persons constituted the 'other'.

By 1947, the International Refugee Organisation (IRO) estimated displaced medical doctor numbers at more than two and a half thousand. This number grew to approximately three thousand by 1949 with renewed movement by doctors mostly from Hungary and Czechoslovakia (Kunz 1975, p. 7). The IRO provided screening for these doctors as many had lost their credentials during the war. Screening was set up in the US zone of Hungary and the British zone of Germany. The story of Robert, born in Germany in 1922, illustrates his experience of Australia through the eyes of a German–Jewish migrant. Robert's father was a medical doctor. When Hitler came to power and life in Germany became extremely dangerous for Jews, he was taken to England by a Quaker organisation; the Movement for the Care of Children. Eventually Robert found himself in Australia and after the war became an Australian citizen. Robert remembers:

> Migrants weren't called "New Australians" in those days. We were refugees- "bloody reffos"
> was the common term-just like some people today say "Wogs" and "Dagoes." On the whole
> Australians were not friendly to migrants. They were so far away from Europe that they had
> no experience of people who came from other cultures; they were intolerant of anyone who
> couldn't speak English. Drunks would abuse you in the trams. Australians didn't even like
> the English much, and "bloody reffos", European Jews, were the end (Lowenstein and Loh
> 1977, p. 57).

Doctors from overseas were required to undertake examinations. Successful doctors received a Certificate of Professional Status and were listed in the Professional Medical Register. The IRO via memorandum approached the Interim Commission of the World Health Organisation (WHO) regarding displaced persons medical practitioners and as a result, a resolution was made. The resolution requested governments to indicate the terms under which these doctors could practise medicine in their countries. Australia's response to this request in 1948 marked the beginning of discriminatory practices which continue to plague IMGs today. The Australian Health Department's response advised the WHO: "under existing conditions, medical practitioners holding only foreign degrees would not be granted registration in Australia to practise their profession" (Kunz 1975, p. 8). Denied registration, doctors from overseas were directed to undergo a minimum of three years of training at Australian medical schools. This was to begin a now common practice, to view IMGs as an underclass through non-acceptance of their qualifications as fully comparable to Australian medical qualifications. There was a growing anti-foreign sentiment in the Australian population, and Australian doctors were no exception.

Widespread anti-foreign rhetoric infiltrated into the ranks of Australian doctors, fuelling their xenophobic non-acceptance of foreign medical practitioners. Most displaced person doctors were specialists and subsequently viewed as a potential threat to Australian trained GPs. Even though displaced person doctors were considered inferior to and less competent than Australian trained doctors, they were sometimes permitted to work in difficult and poorly paid positions. The AMA did not object to some displaced doctors being permitted to work as medical doctors in the Australian Antarctic and in Papua New Guinea. These locations were not attractive to Australian trained doctors and therefore not considered threatening to their livelihoods. So, it seems that perceived inferior overseas trained doctors were not suitable to serve the general Australian population, but were 'good enough' to practise in isolated, desolate places and on black people.

By 1938, there were only four medical schools in Australia (see Lewis 2014) and there was public debate about a shortage of doctors (Committee for the Review of Practices for the Employment of Medical Practitioners in the NSW Health System, 1998, p. 34). Adjustments to restrictions began to emerge. For example, in New South Wales, amendments in 1955 and again in 1957 saw 'preferred' IMGs usually from Commonwealth countries, granted temporary registration in stipulated locations for one year. After five years, full registration was possible. In 1957, the health minister in NSW was empowered to increase the number of doctors seeking 12 months temporary registration. The AMA objected and began a public attack against foreign doctors who were referred to as: "quacks and charlatans and as possessed of what may be termed eastern European standards of ethics" (Iredale 1987, p. 123). A deficit discourse around assumed inferiority of IMG qualifications has a long history. The current rhetoric of the need to maintain high standards and a spirit of livelihood protection can be found back in the 1950s. According to Kamien (2006, p. 3) under persuasion from the AMA, the then NSW Premier wrote to the Prime Minister advocating: "Alien and Refugee Doctors posed an unacceptable competition to Australian doctors who had the highest standards of medical practice in the world". Refugee IMGs are still coming to Australia especially in light of increasing war and terrorism in areas such as the Middle East. Refugee IMGs are qualified medical doctors, a fact Australia seems to resist.

Many refugee doctors have made exceptional contributions to Australian society. For example, Dr Munjed Al Muderis who fled Saddam Hussein's Iraq for fear of execution found himself on a boat from Indonesia, spent time in the now-closed Curtin Detention Centre and eventually became a world-leading osseointegration[3] surgeon (Al Muderis and Weaver 2014). Unfortunately, in view of the Government's current sovereign borders stance on asylum seekers and refugees, a skilled surgeon

---

[3]This surgery involves a pioneering technique that enables amputees to walk again.

such as Dr. Al Muderis, because he arrived in Australia via boat, would never (under any circumstances) be permitted to settle and work in Australia. The institutionalised foundations which underpin this extreme stance can be traced all the way back to 1901 when two significant events occurred: Federation which united Australia's colonies and the White Australia Policy.

## Federation

By the 1880s, many Australians began to identify with Australia as a great nation of brave pioneers rather than a nation with a weakening loyalty to Britain and Empire. A movement for the unification of the Australian colonies began. Hirst (2000, p. 246) argues:

> Federation was in line with British Colonial Office policy, which encouraged the white settler colonies (Canada, New Zealand, South Africa and Australia) to become united, self-governing and self-sufficient 'dominions' within the imperial framework.

In 1901, the Australian colonies which had been settled and developed separately became unified as the Commonwealth of Australia. However, while some argue that in 1901 Australia became a nation state, it is important to highlight that Australia did not have full international sovereignty. Carter (2006, p. 59) points out: "nonetheless 'nationhood', in the form of an imagined community, had been achieved. The nation was imagined both as a united and a *separate* community with a common future-tied to but distinct from Britain's". Australia the nation was 'founded' but it was a nationalist Australia firmly intent on being white and English-speaking (Lueck et al. 2015). The White Australia Policy accompanied Federation.

## The White Australia Policy

The 'new' nation of Australia endorsed by Federation's first Parliament was to be built on a foundation of white race unity. Australia's first peoples were black but that did not seem to pose a problem as it was assumed that the first peoples would die out. Although a few members of Parliament opposed the policy, there was overwhelming community support. Arthur Calwell, first federal minister of Immigration, proposed the Immigration Restriction Act of 1901 (commonly referred to as the White Australia Policy) (Maley 2016). Calwell convinced the Australian public, while war was in recent memory, that a migration programme was necessary for white Australia's protection. Essentially, the policy represented an overt institutionalisation of discrimination, racism and xenophobia. Only Europeans, preferably Northern Europeans, could now immigrate to Australia. The ethnocentric policy therefore implied that the values and beliefs of people with white skin were superior to those of non-whites.

It was assumed that the British Empire would continue its power indefinitely and that white supremacy would always be embedded as valid (Riley 2016). The policy was progressively dismantled between 1949 and 1973.

Historian Henry Reynolds (2003, p. 161) wrote:

> The White Australia policy came to be a source of international embarrassment, a political, moral and intellectual dead-end out of which the nation had with difficulty to negotiate itself while leaving a legacy of suspicion and distrust in the non-European would that continues to the present day.

Xenophobia fuelled the fear of invasion from Asia but there were tragic repercussions for those unwanted peoples already in Australia; Indigenous Australians and South Sea Islanders. The annual visit to Australia's north by the Macassans was banned in 1906. This decision resulted in severed kinship connections and lifelong friendships (Shellam et al. 2017). Some Indigenous Australians found themselves stranded in Indonesia. Many South Sea Islanders were deported resulting in broken marriages and the separation of extended families. The government did not show concern for these traumatic events. Hirst (2014, p. 152) asks: "what made Australians who had little experience of non-Britishers and a good deal of hostility towards them, accept them into their society? The short answer is that the government told them they must". Calwell's appeal: "was not to the benevolence of Australians but to their self-interest, a much more secure basis for policy" (Hirst 2014, p. 153). The ancient land of Australia had evolved into a new nation, a desired homogenous identity of 'the nation'.

## Nationalism

Some historians argue that the true nationalism sentiment in Australia emerged in the ANZAC tradition after the First World War (1914–1918). Garton (2015, p. 124), for example, argues that nationalism in Australia became curiously linked with loyalty to the Empire:

> While nationalism was the ideological glue that held settler societies together in the immediate post war years, preventing social and political disintegration, in Australia these nationalist discourses took on a peculiar character, at once proclaiming the virtues of veterans as founders of the nation while adopting a heightened sense of the importance of ties to the Empire. What emerged was a hybrid discourse that interwove nationalism and Empire loyalism.

The Australian nation today remains reluctant, however, to include and genuinely accept the first Australians. How is it that in the year 2018, 220 years post-invasion, Australia is still unable to come to terms with the idea of a proposed referendum on the recognition of Aboriginal and Torres Strait Islander people in the Australian Constitution? I would argue that this necessary initiative is due to the entrenched xenophobia, ethnocentrism and racism within the Australian nation. Many Australians fear the outsider, the foreign, and many Australians believe that the Australian way, the dominant culture, is a superior one to others. This misbelief began from the early days of the colony and came with the newcomers (Plage et al. 2016). The Eurocentric perception of superiority, however, has ancient roots which run back to Europe which always situated itself apart from the East as its exotic other (Said 1978, 2001). The myth that Europe, Europeans and European ideas were not only superior but the whole of the Western world was also superior infiltrated the new Australian psyche. It seemed that the Eastern world could be totally ignored or discounted as making any worthwhile contribution to humankind. Harding (2011, p. 34) points out:

> Modern European sciences began to emerge in the 16th century. Yet some of the older traditions of China, India and other cultures in Asia and the Middle East were far more sophisticated than European ones until Europe's industrial revolution in the 19th century. It takes a lot of work to create and nourish such Eurocentric ignorance.

Most European Australians by 1900 believed that obtaining national greatness and cohesion was associated with being white and a member of the British race, a race which should not be contaminated by racial interbreeding but rather remain pure. In fact a kind of obsession with the concept of race existed in most Western societies at the time. In terms of Indigenous Australians then, most European Australians held racist views towards the first peoples and this mindset was conveniently expanded to justify the dispossession of Indigenous Australians from their land. In fact according to Markus and Semyonov (2010, p. 2), the dispossession of Indigenous Australians from their lands: "continued well into the twentieth century up until the 1950s and in some cases later". The following 1901 extract from the Bulletin (a prominent nationalistic magazine at that time) provides an example of public sentiment which included the fear of mixed race relations between Indigenous and white Australians:

> If Australia is to be a country fit for our children and their children and their children to live in, we must KEEP THE BREED PURE. The half-caste usually inherits the vices of both races and the virtues of neither. Do you want Australia to be a community of mongrels? (Broom 1994, p. 93).

Indigenous Australians, although considered British subjects, were discriminated against by mainstream society across every Australian institution. As Kleist (2017, p. 192) explains:

> No one experienced the ambivalence of belonging in Australia more than the Indigenous population…they were culturally, legally, and politically excluded until the second half of the twentieth century.

The 1967 referendum gave Australian Indigenous peoples political recognition but not social and cultural belonging (Gunstone 2017). The health system, for example, constituted an exclusion zone for the first people, their descendants and others considered 'non-white'. A white supremacy attitude was extended to the provision or non-provision of medical care. The following is a stark example from Queensland in 1937:

> The committee cannot see its way clear to allow aboriginals and non-whites to be operated on in the theatre nor to receive any surgical after-treatment in the annex to the main building (Hospital committee at Normanton Qld. 1937 in May, 1988, p. 180).

In 1975, the Racial Discrimination Act removed overt racial discrimination from Australian legislation but a residue was left in the treatment of Indigenous Australians and in immigration policies. Moreover, impossible to measure, covert racial discrimination towards Indigenous Australians and migrants remained to lurk in the minds of many white Australians.

Multiculturalism was introduced as a relatively new concept in the 1989 National Agenda for Multicultural Australia. Championed by Labour Prime Minister Paul Keating, multiculturalism was touted as a vision for a better Australia and as the new way forward for the nation. Multiculturalism policy was developed around the three policy objectives of: social justice, the need to nurture a more efficient economy and the maintenance of cultural identity. The imagined Australian community was reframed by the government but was not necessarily accepted by the established Australian community. The policy, as explained by Plage et al. (2016, p. 3):

> Espoused the freedom to maintain distinct cultural heritage and practices, economic efficiency promoted the use of all Australians' skills and social justice incorporated equal opportunities regardless of individual background or ethnicity.

The concept and vision of multiculturalism in modern Australia can however be viewed as problematic as Pettman (1992, p. 8) points out: "The multicultural model may obscure the power of dominant groups and see Australia as a mix of cultures and plurality of interests". Ultimately, the ideal nation state identity sought by Australia was challenged by the rhetoric of multiculturalism. As articulated by Brabazon (1998, p. 60):

> Clearly, there are contradictions between nationalism and multiculturalism. A nation is built on the formation of a fixed, stable citizenry. Migrants will never slot into this nationalist narrative. Their divergent life histories always disrupt the singularity of the nation.

For example, in their 2000 study, Pakulski and Tranter (2000, pp. 217–218) found, eleven years post-multiculturalism, that 'Ethno-nationalists' (those in the Australian population with neo-conservative attitudes) showed:

> Strong preferences for abandoning multiculturalism which is seen as potentially divisive and hindering social adaptation and that it is better if ethnic and racial groups 'blend' into the larger society and do not maintain their distinct traditions and customs, especially if this maintenance occurs with government assistance.

Many Australians remained fearful of the 'other' and protectionist particularly in terms of immigration posing a threat to Australian jobs and as a potential threat to the maintenance of 'Australian' culture. However, Australia still held a desire to cling to Britain and the Commonwealth, with a 1999 proposal to become a republic rejected via a referendum (Gunstone 2017). Australia today remains: "A constitutional monarchy, although interference by the Queen in Australian, as in British politics is virtually unheard of" (Dowding and Martin 2017, p. 60). Australia is often referred to as a young country, for example, in the national anthem: "Australians all let us rejoice for we are young and free". This incongruent situation in mind acclaimed Indigenous opera singer Deborah Cheetham declined an invitation to sing the national anthem at the 2015 Australian Football League grand final and told the media:

> Let me be clear: it was an honour to be asked. The problem is, as an Indigenous leader I simply can no longer sing the words "we are young and free." For that matter, as an Australian with a strong desire to deepen our nation's understanding of identity and our place in the world, I believe we can and must do better (Australian Associated Press 2015).

This objection was also echoed in the behaviour of Indigenous boxer Anthony Mundine, who, before a recent fight (Rothfield 2017), refused to stand for the national anthem. The Australian community, while said to embrace 'fairness' for all, in reality, does not. Rather, the Australian nation is also representative of division and exclusion, and 'fairness' is only the experience for some. Blackshaw (2010, p. 151) succinctly explains:

> Community is always a double. In other words, all its warmth, charm and geniality, notwith-standing, there is much about community that is distinctly unsettling: if one side of its coin is inclusion and harmony, its companion side is always exclusion and oppression.

IMGs in Australia today do not necessarily experience 'fairness'. This book argues that they are othered simply because they are foreign. This chapter has established the development of their current positioning through time. An historical lens has taken the reader from the British invasion in 1788 and the arrival of the first IMGs, British naval surgeons, to the emergence of the imagined Australian nation state of today. The original custodians of the land, Australia's Indigenous peoples, became an ethnic minority in their own country. The scene for subsequent chapters has been set with the flagging of significant historical stages such as Federation, the White Australia Policy and nationalism through to post-war displaced persons and multiculturalism. These aspects of Australian history have significantly influenced and contributed to the state of the nation today. The foundations of the intersecting oppressions of class, race and nation are found in Australia's past. This chapter has established the deliberate long-standing discrimination of IMGs. This is evident in the policies related to the accreditation and registration of IMGs of today and the organisations tasked to administer them. The processes IMGs wishing to work in Australia must engage with are outlined in the following chapter. This enables the reader to appreciate the numerous avenues available and the choices IMGs must make. It is argued that these bureaucratic initiatives are deeply entrenched within the dimensions of structural, hegemonic and interpersonal power.

# References

Al Muderis, M., & Weaver, P. (2014). *Walking free*. Crows Nest: Allen & Unwin.

Arbon, V. (2008). Knowing from where?. In A Gunstone (Ed.), *History, politics and knowledge: Essays in Australian Indigenous Studies* (pp. 134–146). North Melbourne: Australian Scholarly Publishing Pty. Ltd.

Australian Associated Press. (2015). Australia it's time to sing a new song. *Indaily Adelaide Independent*, Tuesday 20 October 2015, Conversation.

Beattie, J. (2016). A case study of chinese migration and colonial development in the british empire, 1860s–1920s. *Environment Modernization and Development in East Asia* (pp. 59–86). Switzerland: Springer.

Blackshaw, T. (2010). *Key concepts in community studies, Sage Key concepts series*. London: Sage Publications.

Blong, K., Kemp, S., & Chen, K. (2016). 'Dating the last major eruption of Long Island, Papua New Guinea: The evidence from Dampier's 1700 voyage on the Roebuck', *Journal Terrae Incognitae: The Journal of the Society for the History of Discoveries, 48*(2), 139–59, viewed 14 May 2017. http://dx.doi.org/10.1080/00822884.2016.1211354.

Brabazon, T. (1998). What's the story morning glory? Perth glory and the imagining of Englishness. *Sporting Traditions, 14*(2), 53–66.

Breen, S. (2008). 'Defending the national honour: The history crusaders and Australia's past'. In A. Gunstone (Ed.), *History, Politics and Knowledge: Essays in Australian Indigenous Studies* (pp. 168–190). Australian Scholarly Publishing Pty. Ltd., North Melbourne.

Broom, R. (1994). *Aboriginal Australians* (2nd ed.). St Leonards, NSW: Allen & Unwin.

Carter, D. (2006). *Dispossession, dreams & diversity: Issues in Australian studies*. Frenchs Forest, NSW: Pearson Education Australia.

Cossart, Y. E. (2014). The Rise and fall of infectious diseases: Australian Perspectives, 1914–2014. *Medical journal of Australia Centenary—History of Australian Medicine, 201*(1), S11–S4. Viewed 14 April 2017, via Medical journal of Australia, www.mja.com.audol:10.5694/mja14.0 0112.

Covacevich, J. (1990). Phangs and physic: 40,000 years of risky business (pp. 61–72). In J. Pearn & M. Cobcroft (Eds.), *Fevers and frontiers*, Queensland: Amphion press, University of Queensland.

Devere, H., Te Maiharoa, K., & Synott, J. P. (Eds.). (2017). *Peacebuilding and the rights of indigenous peoples: Experiences and strategies for the 21st century. The Anthropocene: Politik-economics-society-science*. Switzerland: Springer International.

Doherty, M. (2016). The business of making colonial women visible. *History Australia, 13*(4), 629–631.

Dowding, K., & Martin, A. (2017). Political institutions and policy in Australia. in *Policy Agendas in Australia*. Switzerland: Springer International publishing.

Dunn, M. (2017). *Aboriginal guides in the Hunter Valley, New South Wales, 4*. Switzerland: Springer International, 978–3-319-45011-7 (ebook), http://afes-press-books-de/html/APESS_09.htm.

Etherington, N., & MacKenzie, J.M. (2016). *Exploration and empire*. New Jersey: Wiley, viewed 12 May 2017. https://doi.org/10.1002/9781118455074.wbeoe300, http://onlinelibrary.wiley.com/b ook/doi.org/10.1002/9781118455074.

Garton, S. (2015). Demobilization and empire: Empire nationalism and soldier citizenship in Australia after the First World War—in dominion context. *Journal of Contemporary History, 50*(1), 124–143. Viewed 10 May 2017, https://doi.org/10.1177/0022009414546505, jch.sage.pub.com.

Glynn, I., & Kleist, J. O. (Eds.). (2012). *History memory and migration: Comparisons, challenges and outlooks*. London: Palgrave Macmillan.

Gunstone, A. (2017). Reconciliation, Peace building and Indigenous People in Australia. In H. Devere, K. Te Maiharoa, & J. P. Synott (Eds.), *Peacebuilding and the rights of indigenous people: Experiences and Strategies for the 21st century* (pp. 17–28). Switzerland: Springer International Publishing.

Harding, S. (2011). *The postcolonial science and technology studies reader*. North Carolina: Duke University Press.

Hirst, J. (2000). *The sentimental nation: The making of the Australian Commonmwealth*. Melbourne: Oxford University Press.

Hirst, J. (2014). *Australian history in 7 questions*. Collingwood Vic: Black Inc.

Horton, D. (1996). *AIATSIS map of Indigenous Australia*. Australia: Aboriginal Studies Press.

Hughes, W. (2017). *The economy of the human frame: Phrenology and the nineteenth-century popular imagination*. Manchester: University Press.

Iredale, R. (1987). *Wasted skills: Barriers to migrant entry to occupations in Australia*. Sydney: Ethnic Affairs Commission of New South Wales.

Iredale, R. (2009). Luring overseas trained doctors to Australia: Issues of training, regulating and trading. *International migration, 47*(4), 31–64.

Kamien, M. (2006). OTDs (Overseas trained doctors) and IMGs. Paper presented to Royal Australian College of general practitioners convention, Brisbane, October 7.

Kleist, J. O. (2017). Australia Day from colony to citizenship: 1788–1948 belonging, society and Australia Day. In *Political memories and migration* (pp. 41–101).Basingstoke: Palgrave Macmillan.

Kunz, E. F. (1975). *The intruders: Refugee doctors in Australia*. Canberra: Australian national University Press.

Lawrence, C., & Brown, M. (2016). Quintessentially modern heroes: Surgeons, explorers and empire, c. 1840–1914. *Journal of Social History, 50*(1), 148–178.

Lewis, M. (2014). Medicine in colonial Australia, 1788–1900. *Medical journal of Australia Centenary—History of Australian Medicine, 201*(1), S5–S10, viewed 12 April 2017. http://www.mja.com.au.dol:10.5694/mja14.00153.

Lippmann, L. (1991). *Generations of resistance: Aborigines demand justice* (2nd ed.). Melbourne: Longman Cheshire.

Lowenstein, W. & loh, M. J. (1977). *The immigrants*. Melbourne: Hyland House Publishing.

Lueck, K., Due, C., & Augoustinos, M. (2015). Neoliberalism and Nationalism: Representations of Asylum seekers in the Australian mainstream news media. *Discourse and Society, 26*(5), 608–629. viewed 25 April 2017, https://doi.org/10.1177/0957926515581159, https://www.dasagepub.com.

Maley, W. (2016). Australia's refugee policy: domestic politics and diplomatic consequences. *Australian journal of international affairs, 70*(6), 670–680. viewed 8 November 2016, via Routledge taylor and francis group (Flinders University) http://www.tandfonline.com.exproxy.

Markus, A., & Semyonov, M. (Eds.). (2010). *Immigration and nation building: Australia and Israel Compared. Monash Studies in Global Movements*. Cheltenham, UK: Edward Elgar.

Martyr, P. (2002). *Paradise of quacks: An alternative history of medicine in Australia*. Sydney: Macleay Press.

Maxwell-Stewart, H. (2016). Big data and Australian History. *Australian Historical Studies, 47*(3), 359–364. http://dx.doi.org/10.1080/1031461X.2016.1208728. Via tandfonline.com.

Mcleod, R. (1988). Hamilton of the Pandora: a visiting surgeon in North Queensland. In J. Pearn (Ed.), *Pioneer medicine in Australia* (pp. 57–64). Queensland: Amphion press, University of Queensland.

Muecke, S., & Shoemaker, A. (2004). *Aboriginal Australians: First nations of an ancient continent*. London, UK: Thames & Hudson.

Nettelback, A. (2017). Colonial Protection and the intimacies of Indigenous Governance. *History Australia, 14*(1), 32–47. Viewed 14 May 2017, http://www.tandfonline.com/doi/abs/10.1080/14490854.2017.1286703.

Nugent, M. (2003). Botany bay: voyages, aborigines and history. *Journal of Australian Studies, 27*(76), viewed 17 April 2017, (Taylor and Francis) http://www.tandfoline.com/doi/abs/10.1080/1444.

Pakulski, J., & Tranter, B. (2000). Civic, National and denizen Identity in Australia. *Journal of Sociology, 36*(2), 205–222. Viewed 24 March 2014, via jos.sagepub.com (Flinders University).

Panayi, P. (2016). *Minorities in wartime: National and racial groupings in Europe*. North America and Australia during the two World Wars: Bloomsbury Publishing.

Partington, G. (1998). In those days it was rough: Aboriginal and Torres Strait Islander history and education. In G. Partington (Ed.), *Perspectives on aboriginal and Torres Strait Islander education* (pp. 27–54). Katoomba, NSW: Social science press.

Pearn, J. (1988). First fleet surgeons: A band of brothers disparate. In J. Pearn (Ed.), *Pioneer medicine in Australia* (pp. 33–55). Queensland: Amphion press, University of Queensland.

Pearn, J., & Cobcroft, M. (Eds.). (1990). *Fevers and frontiers*. Queensland: Amphion press, University Queensland.

Pettman, J. (1992). *Living in the margins: Racism, sexism and feminism in Australia*. North Sydney: Allen & Unwin.

Plage, S., Willing, I., Skrbis, Z., & Woodward, I. (2016). Australiannes as fairness: implications for cosmopolitan encounters. *Journal of Sociology, 1*(6), 1–16. viewed 9 February 2017, via Sage (Flinders University, South Australia) http://jos.sagepub.com.

Quigley, K. (2017). Indolence and Illness: Scurvy, the Irish, and early Australia. *Eighteenth-Century Life, 41*(2), 139–153, viewed 16 May 2017, https://doi.org/10.1215/00982601-3841432, http://ecl.dukejournals.org/content/41/2/139.short.

Reid, J. S., Taylor, K., & Hayes, C. (2016). Indigenous health systems and services. In L. Reynolds, H. Keleher, & E. Willis (Eds.), *Understanding the Australian Health Care System* (pp. 153–166). Chatswood: Elsevier.

Reynolds, H. (1987). *The law of the land*, Penguin, Victoria.

Reynolds, H. (2003). *North of Capricorn: The untold story of Australia's north*. Crows Nest: Allen & Unwin.

Reynolds, H. (2013). *Forgotten War*. New South Wales: UNSW Press. Viewed 12 April 2017, (ecite.utas.edu.au) http://www.maristfamily.com.au/resourcedownloads/.

Riley, A. (2016). Same old rhetoric cannot justify banning refugees from Australia. *The conversation*, viewed 17 November 2016. http://www.theconversation.com/same-old-rhetoric-cannot-justify-banning-refugees-from-australia-67923.

Rothfield, P. (2017). *"Anthony Mundine refuses to stand for 'acist' national anthem"*. *Daily Telegraph*, 30 January 2017. Viewed 31 January 2017, https://www.dailytelegraph.com.au/sport/boxing-mma/anthony-mundine.

Said, E. (1978). *Orientalism: Western conceptions of the orient*. London: Penguin.

Said, E. (2001). *Power, politics and culture: Interviews with Edward W.* Said: Pantheon Books, New York.

Shellam, T., Nugent, M., Konishi, S., & Cadzow, A. (Eds.). (2017). *Brokers and boundaries: Colonial exploration in indigenous territory*. Canberra: Australian National University Press and Aboriginal History Inc.

Simpson, R. (1988). John White MD RN surgeon general to the first fleet. In J. Pearn (Ed.), *Pioneer medicine in Australia* (pp. 15–32). Queensland: Amphion press, University of Queensland.

Stanner, W. E. H. (1987). The dreaming. In W. H. Edwards (Ed.), *Traditional aboriginal society* (pp. 225–236). Melbourne: Macmillan.

Steinberg, M. W. (2016). *England's great transformation: law, labor, and the industrial revolution*. Chicago: University of Chicago Press.

Sykes, R. B. (1986). *Incentive, achievement and community: An analysis of black viewpoints on issues relating to black Australian education*. Sydney: Sydney University Press.

Thearle, J. (1990). Complementary medicine: a new frontier. In J. Pearn & M. Cobcroft (Eds.), *Fevers and frontiers* (pp. 117–133). Queensland: Amphion press, University of Queensland.

Van Wyhe, J. (2004). *Phrenology and the origins of Victorian scientific Naturalism, Science Technology and Culture 1700–1945*. England: Ashgate Publishing.

Walker, D. (1999). *Anxious nation: Australia and the rise of Asia 1850–1939*. St Lucia, Queensland: University of Queensland Press.

Woolcock, H. (1988). Medical supervision on nineteenth century emigrant ships: The voyage of the Cliften 1861–1862. In J. Pearn (Ed.), *Pioneer medicine in Australia* (pp. 65–76). Queensland: Amphion Press, University of Queensland.

# Policies, Processes, Poppycock and Dimensions of Power: Structural, Hegemonic and Interpersonal

> For decades, overseas doctors have been faced with a registration system with as many twists and turns as a diseased vascular system (Harris 2011, p. 1).
>
> You start to question whose problem is it? Surely the system cannot be this dysfunctional? The sad fact is it really is! (Dr D, 2012, submission 111).

This chapter configures a framework for an exploration of power and relationships. Dimensions of power are separated and unpacked into categories so that they can be explored in a structured and ordered way. Following the work of Patricia Hill Collins, intersecting oppressions can be organised through a matrix of domination which she explains as: "the overall social organisation within which intersecting oppressions, originate, develop and are contained" (Hill Collins 2000, pp. 228–229).

For this study, three categories are represented: Structural power, hegemonic power and interpersonal power. Structural power refers to the numerous entities that make up the health system and as a result are sanctioned by the government to administer all aspects of health care in Australia. IMGs coming to Australia must engage with the health system as well as various other government departments and agencies. Secondly, hegemonic power probes the Australian medical profession specifically and its power, influence and control as gatekeepers to the health system. The third dimension of power is interpersonal power. This power category is concerned with the voices of IMGs and their relationships and discourses with the system and with the Australian medical profession. The structural power and hegemonic power dimensions have a mutually beneficial role in that they create and maintain the existing power relations. These power relations influence the strategies of control employed by the system to regulate IMGs. This book endeavours to explore the link between macro-analysis of the system and micro-analysis of the individual narratives of IMG experiences. The power differential and relations of power and associated discourses are structured into structural, hegemonic and interpersonal power domains to enable insight into how IMGs are positioned within Australia's medical culture.

© Springer Nature Singapore Pte Ltd. 2019
V. A. Pascoe, *Australia's Toxic Medical Culture*,
https://doi.org/10.1007/978-981-13-2426-0_4

Experiences of coming to Australia, working in Australia, surviving in Australia and the well-being of IMGs in Australia will be explored through the IMG voice, the reflection of lived experience. The complexity of the process journey will be revealed, and the engagement of the doctors within numerous unfamiliar contexts and cultures explored. Ultimately, all relations between the IMG and life in Australia are to a greater or lesser extent mediated by the system. IMG interactions with the deficit discourses of the system are couched in terms of power and oppression.

## Structural Power: The System

The Australian health system is structured in a uniquely national configuration. Belcher (2014, p. 367) suggests that "The Australian health care system can best be described as mixed". There is a distinct public and private sector with both sectors holding responsibility for the provision and delivery of health services to the Australian public. Private practitioners practise their services in public health institutions. They receive payment via a fee-for-service or sessional basis which is funded by a combined contribution of payments from the individuals seeking services, private health insurance providers and government-funded Medicare payments.

The reality of lived experience for IMGs in Australia is controlled by numerous identities within the system. For example, The Medical Board of Australia oversees registration standards. English language tests are administered by several approved providers such as the International English Language Testing System (IELTS). The Australian Medical Council (AMC) controls written medical and clinical examinations. Various Australian medical colleges have their education and training programmes accredited by the AMC. The medical colleges, of which there are sixteen, regulate entry into the specialties. Medicare issues provider numbers, while visas are the domain of the Department of Immigration and Border Protection. This complex bureaucracy, for the sake of simplicity, will be referred to throughout as the system. The system has evolved out of a perceived need to scrutinise, regulate and control IMGs. Over time, the system has managed to escape any major change which could undermine its dominant position and represents an ongoing and seemingly growing power structure. IMGs must undertake a process journey through the requirements of the system through which a power differential is operationalised.

## The Process Journey Through the System

The following information enables the reader to track the process IMGs undertake to begin work as a medical doctor in Australia and therefore gain an appreciation of what is expected of them. It is important to bear in mind here that if an IMG is unsuccessful at any step throughout the process journey, the IMG is required to begin the process journey again from the start.

To gain full Australian medical registration, an IMG must undertake the following: obtain all required documentation for immigration, accreditation and registration purposes. A number of forms specific to the IMGs selected immigration, accreditation and registration pathway must be completed in the exact prescribed format and relevant application fees paid.[1] If any required documentation is not in English, they must arrange for its translation by an approved government-certified interpreter. Documentation must be verified as stipulated in the requirements of the relevant organisation or agency. IMGs must also pass mandatory English language proficiency examinations. If any of the steps required are not undertaken exactly as directed, extra costs will be involved and the application's progress delayed.

For example, according to the National Rural Health Alliance (2011, pp. 12–13):

> If there is a document needing verification that is missing, the OTD will need to ensure that additional documents are signed by the same individual as previously. The complexity of the processes for the application to the AMC is illustrated by the fact that the 'Quick Guide' runs to 72 pages and an additional guide for specialists covers 42 pages.

Extensive requirements can result in lengthy delays in processing applications. This seems at odds with the immediate imperative to facilitate the movement of IMGs into areas of need as quickly as possible. IMGs are not eligible for a Medicare provider number unless they work in a District of Workforce Shortage (DWS). This also applies to overseas graduates from Australian medical schools and Australian trained bonded doctors who agree to be bonded to practise for a period of time in a DWS. A DWS is an area deemed as having below-average access to medical doctors. General practice in inner metropolitan areas of Australian capital cities is classified as non-DWS (apart from Darwin due to its ongoing doctor shortages and remoteness). The classification of areas as DWS was updated as part of the Rural Classification Reform and came into operation on 10 February 2016[2] (DoctorConnect 2016).

The Australian Government, in response to doctor shortages in rural and remote areas of Australia, has initiated an International Recruitment Strategy. According to the Australian Government Department of Health's DoctorConnect website (Commonwealth Department of Health 2016), the first step in the process for an IMG wanting to practise in Australia requires the applying doctor to obtain skill recognition. This is done by visiting the Australian Medical Council website (AMC) (2016) where the doctor needs to choose a registration pathway: competent authority, standard or specialist. The standard pathway can involve either AMC examinations or workplace-based assessment. The specialist assessment pathway leads to full comparability/Area of Need (AON). Area of Need classification is determined by state and territory health authorities (Medical Board of Australia 2016). In addition, the doctor must have medical qualifications verified through primary source verification and meet English language standards. The AMC's role is to assess the: "knowledge, clinical skills and professional attributes of IMGs" (Commonwealth Department of Health 2016). The AMC also assesses applications for recognition of medical specialities. There are two ways to progress identified here, depending on whether or not

---

[1]Fees payable to a specialist college may be as much as $8000.00.

[2]DWS areas listed at DoctorConnect—Home page: http://www.doctorconnect.gov.au/.

the doctor has a job. If the doctor already has a job, he or she is required to apply to the Australian Health Practitioner Regulation Agency (AHPRA) (Australian Health Practitioner Regulation Agency 2016) in the relevant state or territory for registration. Applying doctors are advised that this application may include a pre-employment structured clinical interview (PESCI) assessment of their clinical skills for the job. The next step is to make application to the Department of Immigration and Border Control for a visa and then relocate to Australia. The process of applying to practise medicine in Australia initially seems reasonably straightforward. AHPRA's role is the regulation of Australia's health practitioners, in partnership with and support of the Medical Board of Australia (MBA). The general public can access the AHPRA website for other information such as to check if a medical practitioner is registered or to make a complaint. The MBA is the national board, while there are medical boards supporting the national board in each state and territory. According to the MBA website (2016), the state and territory boards each have several committees such as the: "Registrations committee, health committee, immediate action committee and notifications committee". Not only is the MBA responsible for regulating medical practitioners practising in Australia, which seems to be administered by the supporting body AHPRA, it is also charged with handling complaints, registration renewals and supervision guidelines. In addition, the MBA approves accreditation standards of medical-related courses of study and assesses IMGs who wish to practise (Medical Board of Australia 2016; Rural Health Workforce Australia 2016). There seems to be overlap here between the MBA and the AMC and the distinction between who does what becomes blurred. For example, I was informed on the AMC website (2016) that English language proficiency proof is required by the MBA not the AMC. I was then directed by the MBA website to the AHPRA site for further information. Requirements and processes could easily become unclear for an IMG trying to identify a suitable route through the system.

DoctorConnect (2016) further advises that if the applying doctor does not have a job, he or she should contact a recruitment agency or a Rural Workforce Agency; there are rural workforce agencies across Australia.[3] The Rural Health Workforce Agency is a government-funded initiative to help address the rural doctor shortage through the administration of the International Recruitment Strategy. The agencies can assist with immigration, employment, registration and orientation. In addition, they offer free recruitment services to rural and remote medical practices for: "the complex activities required to recruit an overseas trained doctor" (Rural Health Workforce Australia 2016). The AMC also affords applying general practitioner IMGs or non-specialist hospital IMGs new to Australia, the opportunity to test their skills via a trial examination which can be undertaken online for a fee of $25.00. The examination consists of multiple choice questions apparently set at the level expected from an Australian trained graduating medical student (Australian Medical Council 2016).

---

[3]Health Networks NT, NSW Rural Doctors Network, Health Workforce Qld., Rural Workforce Agency Vic., Rural Doctors Workforce Agency (SA), Rural Recruitment Plus (TAS) and Rural Health West (WA).

At this point, it is perhaps a good idea to return to the major task of an applying IMG, to obtain a visa and choose an appropriate pathway through an approved provider.

It seems that the applying IMG has several options regarding the most appropriate pathway and there are numerous visa categories[4] available to those wanting to live and work in Australia. Some IMGs find the task of selecting an appropriate visa category and/or pathway confusing and time-consuming and, as a result, engage the services of a migration agent or recruitment organisation to assist them. Pathway and visa choices constitute major decisions as these will determine the terms and conditions an IMG will be bound by in Australia. Doctors from New Zealand are in a unique position, however, as most New Zealanders are granted a Special Category Visa (SCV). This visa, while a temporary visa, provides permanent resident status which allows holders to live and work in Australia for an indefinite period. Most other IMGs apply for the Temporary Work (Skilled) Visa (Subclass 457); this visa affords skilled workers the opportunity to work for an approved business for a maximum of four years (Australian Government Department of Immigration and Border Protection 2016). The potential employer is required to formally sponsor the doctor and to provide assurance to immigration authorities that it is unable to fill the position with an Australian citizen or permanent resident who has the necessary skills. The Subclass 457 visa allows an IMG to also bring eligible dependants who too can work or study in Australia. After coming to Australia under this visa, there are no limits on the number of times an IMG and dependants can travel in and out of the country. IMGs who arrived in Australia prior to 26 February 2001 may be able to apply for Australian citizenship; however, if arrival was after 26 February 2001, permanent resident status may need to be achieved first (Australian Government Department of Immigration and Border Protection 2016). Assuming that all goes well for an IMG and a visa is granted from the Department of Immigration and Border Protection, the next complex task is to identify and apply for a pathway.

## Down the Garden Path

Before applying for admission to a pathway and seeking registration in any category, IMGs must have their primary sources verified via the approved AMC process. Verification of qualifications is mandated under the Health Practitioner Regulation National Law Act 2009 (Australian Medical Council 2016). From October 2015 The International Credentials Services of the Educational Commission for Foreign Medical Graduates' (ECFMGs) Electronic Portfolio of International Credentials (EPIC) conducts verification (Educational Commission for Foreign Medical Graduates 2016). The results are uploaded to the AMC's qualifications portal. The portal is used by the MBA for registration process and by the specialist colleges for assessment purposes. This initiative seems like a streamlining process. This may be however a frustrating

---

[4]For the full range of visas see the Department of Immigration and Border Protection at https://www.border.gov.au/trav/check-your-visa-and-work-entitlements,andImmigrationdirect.com.au.

or even terminating experience for some IMGs as the AMC website (2016) provides a list of overseas institutions that are often slow to respond to the request or unfortunately do not respond at all! If qualifications cannot be verified, a doctor's application cannot proceed.

The MBA (Medical Board of Australia 2016) outlines the options for an IMG as follows:

## The Competent Authority Pathway

IMG applicants must have successfully completed a bachelor of Medicine and Surgery from an AMC and World Directory of Medical Schools (WDOMS)-approved institution in: the UK, Canada, the USA, New Zealand or Ireland (World Directory of Medical Schools 2016). IMGs from other countries are excluded. If doctors meeting these requirements have also obtained employment, they may apply to the MBA for provisional registration. After satisfactory completion of twelve months (or a minimum of 47 weeks full time) of practice under supervision, IMGs in this pathway may become eligible to apply to the MBA for general registration. Eligibility for this pathway does not guarantee an IMG smooth and timely progress to registration, however, and some become so discouraged that they give up trying. In their submission to the 2012 Parliamentary Inquiry, the National Rural Health Alliance (2011, submission 113, p. 11) gave the following example to the 2012 committee:

> Dr G is an Irish born and qualified GP with the appropriate qualifications to be categorised as eligible for mutual recognition by the RACGP. She therefore represents those OTDs with the easiest pathway to registration as she is substantially comparable to an Australian GP specialist. In early 2010 she moved to Australia with her husband who has a clinical fellowship in a large teaching hospital. She recently decided to start working as a GP, and was able to find a position in an outer metropolitan practice with District of Workforce Shortage (DWS) status. Although she already had the relevant visas to allow her to work in Australia, she was required to complete over twenty different forms, pay approximately $3500 in various fees and comply with a variety of additional requirements. It has been five months since she first applied for the specialist pathway with the AMC and she is still not registered to practise.

Needless to say, the submission further notes that the doctor in question has stated that she will not be encouraging her colleagues and friends in Ireland to consider seeking work in Australia.

## The Standard Pathway

This pathway is suitable for IMGs who are not eligible for the competent authority pathway or specialist pathway and are seeking general registration with the MBA. To be considered for this pathway however doctors need to apply directly to the

AMC. This pathway requires the IMG to pass the AMC multiple choice and clinical examinations. If both examinations are passed prior to making application to the MBA for registration, the applicant can apply for limited registration. Most applicants are assessed through this method. There is also the option for standard pathway (workplace-based assessment). In this case, the doctor must pass the AMC multiple choice examination and have his or her clinical skills and knowledge assessed in the workplace. The IMG must complete twelve months of supervised practice or a minimum of forty-seven weeks full-time service in an approved position. The MBA (2016) notes that few IMGs are assessed this way as there are limited numbers of approved assessment programmes (only 7 locations across Australia). If IMGs taking this pathway have passed the AMC multiple choice and clinical examinations before beginning supervised practice, they may make application for provisional registration. IMGs may work under supervision in general practice positions or hospital positions. In addition, IMGs may be directed to undertake the pre-employment structured clinical interview (PESCI) before applying for limited or provisional registration.

In an effort to be clearer regarding registration categories, they are summarised below from the MBA (2016):

## Seeking Limited Registration

Before applying for limited registration, an IMG must have obtained an offer of employment and have passed the AMC multiple choice examination. The limited registration is linked to the position; for example, an IMG may be granted limited registration for postgraduate training or supervised practice. Limited registration may be granted for work if it is located in an Area of Need (AON).

To clarify, DoctorConnect (2016) advises that an Area of Need (AON) is determined by state or territory governments for immigration and registration purposes as opposed to a District of Workforce Shortage (DWS) which is determined by the Department of Health for the purposes of access to Medicare. DoctorConnect (2016) further advises that an employer wishing to gain approval to employ an IMG, in most cases, will need to meet both AON and DWS status.

## Provisional Registration

To be considered for provisional registration, an IMG must pass the AMC multiple choice and clinical examinations (AMC certificate holders). Provisional registration requires the IMG to have obtained employment.

## General Registration

IMGs on the standard pathway complete twelve-month supervised practice (minimum of forty-seven weeks full-time service) in an approved position before they become eligible to apply for general registration.

## English Language Proficiency

The AMC (2016) advises IMGs to make arrangements to provide proof of English language proficiency (ELP) before applying to enter any assessment pathway. IMGs may also apply for an exemption from the ELP requirement. Of particular interest here is a statement from the MBA (2016, p. 4): "The board reserves the right at any time to revoke an exemption and/or require an applicant to undertake a specified English language test". The board notes that the ELP standards were last reviewed 1 July 2015 and that review is undertaken at least every 3 years.

The specialist medical colleges offer various pathways for IMGs, and once an IMG has moved through the other processes, a specialist medical college needs to be selected for the IMG to progress through to full recognition in his or her speciality area of expertise. For example, the DoctorConnect website (2016) advises that the Australian College of Rural and Remote Medicine (ACRRM) has an IMG programme. The ACRRM website (2016) states that it is the only college in the world to offer a speciality in rural and remote medicine. ACRRM's programme leads to general registration, and a specialist pathway leads to registration in a relevant speciality.

The AMC (2016) advises that specialist pathway recognition applications must go directly to one of the sixteen medical colleges. Following qualification verification from ECFMG's Electronic Portfolio of International Credentials, the applicant is directed to go online to the AMC to set up an AMC portfolio. The relevant college assesses the comparability of the applicant against what is expected for an Australian trained specialist in the same field of practice. Once all requirements have been satisfied and assessment has been successfully completed, the IMG can apply for the pathway Specialist Recognition or Area of Need. The applicant must apply to the MBA for registration. The MBA (2016) advises that the colleges will assess IMGs as: not comparable or, substantially comparable or, partially comparable (there does not seem to be a fully comparable category) and that the IMG "may be required to undertake a period of peer review (oversight) which may involve completion of workplace-based assessment or a period of supervised practice and further training, which may involve college assessment, including examinations". The MBA (2016) confirms the requirements of the specialist pathway—Area of Need (as at 1 October 2015), as a pathway which does not lead to specialist registration but the applicant can also apply for specialist pathway—Specialist Recognition if seeking specialist registration with the MBA. The IMG is able to complete the requirements for Specialist Recognition at the same time as working in an AON. The IMG is assessed by the college for suitability to the position identified by the employer. The employer must demonstrate that the position cannot be filled, and as a result, there is an "adverse impact on service delivery". (Medical Board of Australia 2016). The employer then selects a suitable AON application to the position (the applicant must be eligible to apply to the MBA for limited Registration AON).

It is beyond the scope of this book to explore all possible processes for each speciality college. ACRRM's pathways represent a unique proposition. ACRRM is accredited by the AMC for the speciality of General Practice (dedicated to rural and remote practice). The ACRRM website (2016) notes that both the workplace-based assessment and the competent authority programmes offered by the college closed in July 2014. These pathways now sit with the MBA in an effort to minimise duplication and work towards streamlining processes as recommended by the 2012 Parliamentary Inquiry Report. ACRRM provides the following options for IMGs:

## Standard Pathway

This pathway is for a non-specialist IMG and leads to registration. ACRRM (2016) has AMC approval in each state and territory to conduct pre-employment structured clinical interview (PESCI) assessment. Applicants to the standard pathway are required to undertake a PESCI. If the IMG has successfully completed assessment, gained registration and completed twelve months of medical practice in Australia, he or she may be eligible to train for fellowship of ACRRM via the Independent Pathway.

## Independent Pathway

This pathway is solely owned and administered by the college. It is designed for experienced doctors who require "self-directed learning and flexibility" (ACRRM 2016). IMGs are invited to apply after undertaking a process of recognition of prior learning (RPL).

## Specialist Pathway

An IMG may be eligible to obtain Fellowship of ACRRM (FACRRM) if he or she has college recognised general practice specialist qualifications. The college states: "this pathway is a fair and equitable pathway for IMGs to achieve FACRRM specialist medical registration in Australia and vocational recognition" (ACRRM 2016). Perhaps pathways offered elsewhere do not offer a fair and equitable pathway?

Applicants must have skills and expertise that are considered substantially or partially comparable to those of an Australian trained fellow of the college and have overseas general practice qualifications as identified in the college's codified list.[5] This pathway enables doctors to practise independently anywhere within Australia.

The above represents only a thumbnail sketch of the process journey through the system and all its possibilities. The devil seems to be in the detail because attached to all these processes are the micro-interactions between IMGs and the system, the small steps which need to be taken between and through the broader framework presented here. How do they navigate their way within such a powerful structure with firmly institutionalised ways of doing business?

IMGs are individual actors, not a homogeneous group. Rather, they come from diverse cultural backgrounds and have a range of different life experiences, norms, values and aspirations. The IMG experience in the system is also an individual journey. Some IMGs seem to have a reasonable relationship with the system, while others report their relationship as problematic, even horrendous. IMGs however share an occupation, and they constitute a professional group, that of medical doctors. As a professional group, they also share the fact that they obtained their basic medical training in a country other than Australia. As a group of overseas trained medical practitioners, IMGs have a dedicated group position in the system, that of the other, an inferior position assigned to them by the system. IMGs somehow, even though they are also medical doctors, do not quite belong in the Australian medical profession. Initially, their overseas qualifications are often presumed as lacking or deficient in some way and consequently can be treated as inferior to those of Australian trained doctors. For example, the following experience of an IMG GP participant in Hawthorne, Birrell and Young's study conducted in regional Victoria (2004, pp. 41–42):

> Truly (peer relationships are) a difficult area because I don't feel that I'm really accepted. I feel that other doctors are not happy. I feel that my patients, they really like me. A lot of patients, they're glad to see me. But I don't feel accepted by other doctors. Definitely I have a lot of problems with other doctors in the Clinic, little problems because in many situations I just let go because it's no point arguing and making more tension in the Clinic. In the first few months I wasn't given the key to the front door, I was kept outside with the patients until it was time to get in. Then I was given the key only to one lock, so I can't get into the Clinic after hours. I don't feel that I'm trusted.

IMGs must prove themselves (in some cases continually) to the system. However, even if an IMG is able to satisfy the numerous requirements of the system, he or she is not necessarily entitled to leave the other status group and become a fully fledged member of the Australian trained medical doctor group. From the very beginning of the process journey, the IMG/system relationship is couched in a 'deficit' discourse and this often continues throughout the process journey. According to the Australian Doctors Trained Overseas Association (ADTOA): … "the professional and personal

---

[5]The list mentions eligible awards and institutions from the following countries only: Belgium, Canada, Denmark, Hong Kong, Ireland, Netherlands, New Zealand, Norway, Singapore, South Africa, Sweden, UK and USA.

lives of hard working IMG doctors are being destroyed by this dysfunctional and evil system. Rural and regional Australians are literally paying with their lives" (2012). Many remote, rural and regional Australian communities are left with inadequate provision of medical services due to a health workforce shortage. IMGs are recruited to fill the gaps, but many experience difficulties associated with the system. IMGs like Australian trained doctors are medical professionals, and one would think that everything possible would be put in place to expedite the establishment of IMGs in these needy locations.

Moreover, it becomes evident in the following chapter five that the toxic culture within the medical profession in Australia does not always act honestly, in good faith, or put patients' interests first. Many medical professionals including IMGs experience harassment and bullying within Australia's medical culture. Not only do IMGs have to navigate their way through the organisations of the system and their processes, but the requirements can be different. Requirements for individual IMGs can be based on their particular speciality, which country they are from and which visa they have. In addition, the processes are also influenced by the position they obtain and where in Australia the position is located.

The registration processes for IMGs wishing to practise in Australia are arduous and confusing. The final report from the Parliamentary Inquiry Committee (2012) into the registration process for IMGs indicates the state of affairs by its title: "Lost in the Labyrinth". The report notes that while individual bodies within the system may be able to clearly detail their processes, when they combine to become the system as a whole it resembles 'spaghetti' (2012, p. 6). Psychiatrist Dr Llewellyn, medical manager of a regional health district, referred to the registration process as: "bordering on what I see as criminal in its inefficiency" (Hyland 2011). The system is not a seamless entity, and it does not necessarily share information across its various stakeholders.

The system is the vehicle for a powerful interest group that of the medical profession. This high-status group is tasked by the government to direct and police the accepted level of medical care and the required health behaviours of the population. Moreover, they are the expert body with the knowledge to set the requirements for medical training. The qualifications of IMGs are measured against the Australian standards. This in itself is necessary to ensure that standards are met and maintained. However, power relations enter into the equation, and in an effort to keep standards high, the system has evolved into a cumbersome, overzealous maze which only serves to divide medical practitioners into two groups: Australian trained and overseas trained. As a result, many IMGs become trapped and oppressed with some unable to practise medicine at all. Many IMGs feel that their relationship with the system is one of constant struggle and that they are literally fighting the system.

> It seems to me that the real political task in a society such as ours is to criticise the working of institutions which appear to be both neutral and independent; to criticise them in such a manner that the political violence which has always exercised itself obscurely through them will be unmasked, so that one can fight them (Foucault in Rabinow 1984, p. 6).

The process journey for IMGs in Australia is one of the most difficult in the world. According to Stanley, a director of a medical recruitment company quoted in an Age

Newspaper article entitled: Foreign doctors' obstacle course 'a disgrace': "Other Western countries have complex and strict systems, but we (Australia) have the worst system for co-ordination, with a reputation for causing frustration that makes us look ridiculous" (Hyland 2011). Yet, Australia is experiencing a health workforce shortage and IMGs are needed to fill gaps, particularly in rural and remote areas. There seems to be a problem here, and while aspects of this have been acknowledged by various governments, agencies and inquiries, the problem remains largely unaddressed.

The power of the Australian medical profession cannot be underestimated as medical dominance has a gatekeeper role to the Australian health system. The high-status profession of medicine is akin to a ruling class in the health system and is underpinned by a hierarchy of power, self-interest and authority.

## Hegemonic Negotiation: The Australian Medical Profession

Hegemonic negotiation is activated in the Australian medical profession specifically and its power, influence and control as gatekeepers to the health system. The concept of hegemony can be understood in terms of Marx's work on historical materialism where the ruling class (in this case the Australian medical profession) interests are represented as universal interests (in this case the interests of society as a whole). Globally, medicine dominates every aspect of health policy and health delivery (Germov 2005, 2014). In Australia too health policy and health delivery are the domain of the Australian medical profession. Western medical practice in Australia post the 1788 invasion was closely linked to the British practice of medicine. In fact, the Australian Medical Association (AMA) was not formed until 1962, before then, medical doctors in Australia were represented by the British Medical Association. Keleher (2016, p. 397) argues that:

> Both organisations have actively worked to ensure that the State is removed from regulating the private practice of doctors apart from the funding of registration bodies. The medical profession has nurtured the State through sophisticated advocacy to ensure the institutionalisation of medical power.

The AMA is a powerful body and constitutes the primary professional body for the medical profession, it has a reported membership of approximately 27,000 (2015). There are also other bodies that represent medical doctors such as the Australian Doctors Trained Overseas Association (ADTOA) which gives advocacy and representation to IMGs; however, it is not anywhere near as powerful as the AMA. The AMA: … "actively lobbies governments, fiercely defends fee-for-service medicine and has a strong focus on industrial issues" (Keleher 2016, p. 400). Medical dominance has always operated to a degree in the Australian health context. The economy and the state play a role in the maintenance of medical dominance (Keleher 2016; Willis 2006). Governments support medical dominance because they are responsible for the health and welfare of the population; as a result, governments endorse and value the expert knowledge and advice of the medical profession. The work of

Foucault is particularly helpful in the analysis of medicine and associated issues as his approach is systematic and can be applied to medical institutions, to the body and to governmentality (Hodges et al. 2014; Turner 1995). Foucault's (1991, p. 102) development of what he terms 'governmentality' defines the structure and function of governments as:

> the ensemble formed by the institutions, procedures, analyses and reflections, the calculations and tactics that allow the exercise of this very specific albeit complex form of power, which has as its target population, as its principal form of knowledge political economy, and as its essential technical means apparatuses of security.

It was in the second half of the eighteenth century Foucault argued that politics and the focus of governments shifted from concerns of the individual to the needs and welfare of populations as a whole (Crampton and Elden 2016). Foucault explored relationships in society between discourses and power, according to Turner (1995, p. 10) particularly in relation to medicine: "that is the development of alliances between discourse, practice and professional groups". Foucault's work is not only complex and open to many different interpretations but has also shifted over time (Gariepy 2016). Nevertheless as stated by Zamora (2016, p. 2): "His ideas have been used in fields as diverse as history, philosophy, anthropology, political science, sociology, gender studies and post-colonial studies". Many of Foucault's classic works on key concepts such as 'power', 'discipline' and 'governmentality' are the focus of scholars today, McCall (2016, p. 52) suggests: "as they attempt to make sense of our neoliberal present" Dawes (2016) while endorsing Foucault's works with the potential for deeper analysis of liberalism and neoliberalism, notes that scholars often do not explain the concept. In acknowledgement of that omission, it has been described as a 'new' capitalism or the global economy and its innate inequalities. Usually, explanations include factors such as an onus on individual responsibility, privatisation, free trade and markets and the restriction of State intervention (Nguyen 2017). Dawes (2016, p. 286) offers a broader description:

> Neoliberalism is seen as the reinvention of the classical liberal tradition, expanded to encompass the whole of human existence, whereby the market stands as the ultimate arbiter of truth, and where freedom is recoded to mean anything the market allows.

Foucault's critical attitude explored liberalism as a part of a form of complex government rationality and he believed it should be approached: "Neither as 'an ideal' that one should devote oneself to, nor as an 'ideology' that can simply be exposed and opposed" (Raffnsoe et al. 2016, p. 290). For Foucault, the market became the point of reference for liberalism. According to Betta (2016), the free market, economic interest, and the self-regulating forces of the market became the substance of liberalism. For Foucault: "the liberal government and its capitalist system needed freedom. It consumed freedom, which means it must produce it, it must organise it" (Betta 2016, p. 31–32). Lorenzini (2016, p. 46), states that according to Foucault: "freedom is not a metaphysical concept: on the contrary, the exercise of freedom is always punctual and relative to a certain given configuration of power relations". The rise of clinical medicine was also of interest to Foucault. In his work entitled:

"The Birth of the Clinic" (2003) he explored the power and control of medicine, the development of the clinical gaze and how knowledge gains legitimisation (Hodges et al. 2014; McCall 2016). Foucault took a particular interest in psychology and psychiatry (which he considered a 'dubious science' (Powell 2015) and the distinction between the 'mad' and the 'sane' where, at a time when 'madness' and 'illness' were linked, he claimed that the 'sane' held moral control over the 'mad' (Ninnis 2016).

Foucault maintained that the human body itself represents a station for circulating relations of power and that rule of the human body underpins professional regimes of power. Powell (2015, p. 409) further argues: "Indeed, the success of modernity's domination over efficient bodies in industry, docile bodies in prisons, patient bodies in clinical research and regimented bodies in schools and residential centres attest to Foucault's thesis". Another two critical areas of Foucault's work embrace concerns of genealogy and the archives of knowledge.

Foucault was an advocate of the historical perspective of Genealogy which encourages investigation to assist critique of how the present has been crafted by the past, to reveal the relationship between knowledge, power and the human subject. Genealogy then, as advanced by Wang (2017, p. 2):

> Seeks to illuminate the contingency of the taken for granted, to denaturalise what seems immutable, to destabilise seemingly natural categories as constructs and confines articulated by discourse, opening up new possibilities for the future.

Hand in hand with genealogy is Foucault's notion of an Archaeology of Knowledge. Archaeology seeks to investigate the history of the structures within society which have created and moulded the boundaries around ideas, knowledge and truth; subsequently revealing representations and discursive formations (Hanson and Ogunade 2016). Linked to historical notions of truth, knowledge, rationality and the need for contextualisation:

> Foucault's archaeology examined the conditions of emergence, how and why a given society/era recognises certain things as knowledge, how and why some procedures are considered rational and others not (Wang 2017, p. 2).

As a result, if deemed irrational, individuals and groups may become marginalised or excluded. Foucault, was a supporter of marginalised groups and pro civil society, his term 'totalising institutions' referred to the centralising of power and he was interested in the effects that follow when totalising institutions monopolise knowledge (Nica 2017; Villadsen 2016). For Raffnsoe et al. (2016), Foucault's investigations of knowledge and government have become reflected in today's working and private life, regardless of where an individual is situated in the social order; marginalised or at its centre.

Discursive and non-discursive practices create the agenda and exercise powerful influence. A discursively constituted effect of power becomes truth which subsequently grants legitimacy to specialised forms of knowledge, which then reinforce and reproduce power (Gordon 1980; Legg 2016). Moreover, Legg (2016, p. 860) asserts that: "It is the command to tell and know the truth, that Foucault suggests, marks the intimate intrusion of governmentality into self-conduct". Over time, Foucault became increasingly interested in the self and interaction between the self and others. According to Depew (2016), Foucault noted that perhaps in the past he focussed too much on technologies of power and domination and not enough on technologies of individual domination and power relations. That is, the chosen action taken by an individual upon his or herself by way of the technologies of the self (Tazzioli 2016). In fact, Foucault claimed that: "the conduct of oneself is one of the best aids for coming to terms with the specificity of power relations" (Depew 2016, pp 28–29). Ultimately, for Foucault, the Platonic Model espouses that truth results from self-knowledge (Cohen 2017; Peters 2017). Explained by Depew (2016, p. 28): "The relation between the reflexivity of the self, on the self, and the knowledge of the truth is established in the form of the already-there, and self-knowledge is arrived at in the element of identity". Foucauldian ideas, according to Zamora (2016, p. 2) have become: "a central intellectual reference of our time". Hampton (2016, p.115), in discussion of the marginal role given to the humanist tradition within Foucault's work on power, suggests why:

> In the decades since his death (1984), many of the great humanist themes: the ethics of governments, the spatial expansion of empire, the dynamics of migration and diaspora – have made their return. In a global culture, the intersection between ethical government, spatial practice, and the movement of populations persists as a post-antihumanist concern.

In a global culture, medical migration is a constant (Bonditti et al. 2017). IMGs continue to choose Australia as a preferred country in which to practise medicine. Once in Australia IMGs are confronted with a medical profession based on a hierarchy of power, authority and self-interest. The pursuit of self-interest is linked to the exercise of power as Depew (2016, p. 26) confirms: "If an individual seeks to gain political power over others, one cannot transform one's privileges into political action on others, into rational action, if one is not concerned about oneself". Foucault's systematic approach offers a useful lens through which to view medical dominance and the ramifications of its actions and behaviours. The historical perspective applied to the rise of the medical profession and the development of the supporting structures and process which underpin it are illuminated by Foucault's complimentary concepts of Genealogy and the Archaeology of Knowledge. Knowledge shapes action taken and power exercised which in turn, shape new knowledge and its assigned credibility. Over time legitimacy of what is truth is established.

Powell (2015, p. 403) explains:

> Other interpretations are simultaneously discounted and delegitimised. The result is a view and mode of practice in which power and knowledge support each other. These domains not only sustain, for example, certain professional discourses, they mould what those professions might become.

The expert knowledge of the medical profession in Australia has been granted legitimacy by the government and as a result, assumes a powerful superior status over other health professionals. The beginnings of the professions can be located as long ago as the eleventh century when craftspeople (such as bakers and cobblers) of the same trade formed associations. These early associations are similar to modern associations today. According to Susskind and Susskind (2015, p. 20):

They came together to set standards, control competition, to look after the interests of their members and families, and to enjoy the prestige of being part of a group of recognised experts.

Contemporary professions developed especially in the nineteenth century with the rise of capitalism and other scholars of the time had varying perspectives on how to view the professions. For example, for Durkheim they were a vehicle for integration and regulation in modern society and constituted a move away from excessive individualism. Weber was able to include their rise in his ideas of class and market economy where there was increasing rationalisation and bureaucratisation in society. Functionalist, Talcott Parsons stressed the function of the professions as a positive for modern society in terms of the maintenance of social order. On the other hand, the professions and professionalism viewed from a conflict perspective represented vehicles for power, authority and control. "Since British colonisation, medicine in Australia has developed as a strong market-based industry" (Keleher 2016, p. 397). By 1880, Willis (1989, p. 60) argues:

Medicine had a high-status, reasonably politically effective vanguard elite who utilised their class positions and contacts in the political sphere to further the cause of the occupation as a whole (the external dynamic) while attempting to regulate and reform it from within (the internal dynamic).

The medical profession is male-dominated despite the fact that the number of female graduates is now equal to males. According to the Australian Institute of Health and Welfare (2015), women constitute 38.6%, nearly two in five of all doctors. The medical profession's population represents an ageing workforce however with the average age of male doctors at 48 years and the average age of female doctors at 41 years. Women are underrepresented in the surgical fields. Nevertheless, the Australian population endorse the medical profession to be the custodians of population health.

How are IMGs placed within the profession and what does the Australian trained medical profession and the system expect from them? Importantly why are they placed as they are; a professional underclass within an elite profession? Turner (1995, p. 133) argues that professionalisation itself can be regarded as a strategy of occupational control which "structures the relationship between experts, patrons and clients" (see Powell 2015; Susskind and Susskind 2015). In terms of IMGs, the system has developed a number of strategies for control which conspire to limit, regulate and exclude IMGs so that their marginalisation is maximised. Strategies of control include such measures as examinations and fees.

## Strategies of Control—Examinations

Australia has a long history of exclusionary practices and assessment methods directed towards overseas trained medical practitioners. For example, after the Second World War when displaced person medical doctors came to Australia hoping for a new life and the opportunity to utilise their medical skills, they were met with discriminatory policies and strategies. A shocking practice is mentioned by Iredale (2009, p. 44): "Sydney University was notorious. It took 'refugee doctors' for retraining but right up till 1974 it only allowed eight to graduate each year. If more qualified, a ballot was held". Another illuminating example from much later in 1998 shows that inquiries are not able to make any real changing impact on the discriminatory practices. Marked differences were found in the assessment of Australian medical students and AMC candidates. The NSW Committee for Review of Employment (1998) found that this impeded not only the chances of AMC candidates from obtaining the required standard but also their access to employment. The Committee recommended (1998) that: "to ensure procedural fairness and to avoid complaints of discrimination, the Australian Medical Council examinations be based on a clearly articulated curriculum" (Iredale 2009, p. 46). Assessment within Australian medicine, while deemed essential in the interests of maintaining high standards, can become a vehicle for exclusion.

The system controls the entry of overseas trained medical professionals into the Australian health system via examinations and assessments that are difficult to access, attract fees and have lengthy delays. Some IMGs do not pass both examinations; for example, a doctor may pass the AMC multiple choice examination but fail the clinical examination. As a result, some IMGs are required to resit examinations sometimes many times. Dr Iredale has worked on issues associated with IMGs for over thirty years and made a submission to the 2012 Parliamentary Inquiry, in her view:

> The AMC exams are an example of systemic discrimination where certain ethnic/linguistic (NESB) groups do not achieve pass rates comparable to ESB groups. In countries like the US, this would require the AMC to prove that the exams are not discriminatory. In Australia, however, differential rates are attributed to the lesser knowledge and skills of certain candidates (2012, submission 134, p. 5).

Strategies for control are developed and operationalised as if IMGs represented an alternate form of healthcare professionals. The system seems to regard and treat IMGs in the same way as it does other allied health bodies, that is the need to control them, establish boundaries around them and do the utmost to if not exclude them, at least marginalise them (Twohig 2016). Could it be that IMGs are perceived by the system to constitute a type of alternative care or even competition? Perhaps the situation for IMGs can be seen in these terms:

> Professionalism restricts entry into the medical market place which is controlled by professional associations via a system of formal exams. Professional medicine attempts to regulate the market to prevent the introduction of alternative systems of care. These controls on entry bring about limitations on competition…There is little public regulation of prices and the supply of service because of the existence of medical dominance (Turner 1995, p. 195).

Examinations carry with them a great deal of power, the power to grant acceptance and the power to fail (McCall 2016). For IMGs particularly, unsuccessful examination results can result in costly resit fees or even be career ending. Found in all mechanisms of discipline, Foucault described examinations as:

A constantly repeated ritual of power. The examination combines the techniques of an observing hierarchy and those of a normalizing judgment. It is a normalizing gaze, a surveillance that makes it possible to qualify, to classify, and to punish. It establishes over individuals a visibility through which one differentiates them and judges them (Rabinow 1984, p. 197).

At a public hearing conducted by the 2012 Parliamentary Inquiry, it was noted that an IMG had waited more than a year to even obtain a place in a clinical examination (Harris 2011). Dr. W highlights the lengthy waiting time IMGs can experience:

After passing the AMC MCQ examination, the average wait for a position in the clinical AMC examination is 18 (!) months which exacerbates doctors' "time out of clinical work." There are no explanations why some IMGs have to wait much longer than 18 months!!! It gets worse for IMGs who fail in their first attempt, they face a wait of about 22 months, in some cases even up to 3 years! The situation is compounded by the AMC conducing unlimited MCQ examinations locally and overseas at a time where they cannot provide AMC clinical examination positions within a reasonable time! (2012, submission 68, p. 2).

In our interview, Alex expressed his opinion of examinations for IMGs in Australia believing that IMGs are given false information about the level required:

They say they are at intern level but they are not, they are much harder than that. When too many of us start passing they make the exam even harder (2012, interview 10).

In Dr. G's opinion, examination fees are very expensive and pose a particular difficulty for those IMGs who come from poor countries, while for the bureaucracy, fees represent a good source of earning:

To get fully registered an OTD has to pay through the nose to sit exams and to prepare for them. Since most of the candidates are from poor countries - where would they get the money from? There is quite an industry based on such a necessity. Exams are hideously expensive. Every time there is a failure, it has to be repeated. Nice little earner (2012, submission 31 p. 2).

Dr. A, after more than five years of exemplary service, was suddenly required to sit an examination:

The College and AOA (Australian Orthopaedic Association) have assessed my qualification and experience before I immigrated to Australia. They have found me suitably qualified and trained to work as an Orthopaedic surgeon in an AON position in X. Even though I have filled this position for more than five years and performed to the upmost satisfaction of my employing Health Service and to standards of the College, I am now compelled to verify my competency in an Exam usually taken at entry to the profession. This doesn't make any sense. I was allowed to perform thousands of operations and had in excess of ten thousand patient appointments. My surgical practice is audited, peer reviewed and surgical outcomes are documented, easily comparing to Australian and International standards. Why is it that now a different set of rules applies to grant me unconditional registration or at least a location specific, not time limited registration to continue my work in X? (2012, submission 66).

Dr. BJ's clinical examination experience is almost unbelievable. It was a difficult examination experience anyway due to interruption and criticisms from examiners regarding his English but imagine Dr. BJ's surprise when his feedback letter arrived:

The female patient of my second long case was replaced by a male patient. I was really confused about a male patient who could have a past history of total hysterectomy and mastectomy. Perhaps it can only be diagnosed by Australian trained physician in Australia, who is also an examiner for the FRACP clinical examination (2012, submission 26).

Many IMGs find the examination preparation and access process a very stressful time particularly as so much is at stake, their capacity to work in their profession in a new country. Failure can result in loss of income, adverse impacts on family life and ongoing pressure. Examinations constitute an exclusionary practice (those who pass and those who do not); this has a potentially disempowering influence on an IMG's self-esteem. A participant in Hawthorne et al.'s study (2004, p. 46) spoke of examination failure and the associated pressures:

I've written the Fellowship twice and I've failed it and I can see why, because I was not prepared for it. I will not speak for all the South Africans, but the outlook there was a bit different from Australia. The first time I looked for help, but there was no help. So I went to write it again and I made exactly the same mistakes. But still they have this hammer over your head and say, "Pass or you can't carry on with the five-year plan." I see myself very much as an Australian doctor but I think after such hardships it's very difficult to go to exams, and I never, ever, ever failed an exam before. I have three degrees - I went through them quite easily. Now my colleagues said, if they don't like the way that you do it, you might never get this exam. Someone at the College said to me, "Oh we're confident you will eventually pass it." And the word 'eventually' is a terrible thing.

For Schroder and Thompson (2015) the ethical dimension of examinations and the relation to self is of particular concern. "The praxis of examination entails self-confrontation in the light of the uncertainty regarding that which is expected of the self". IMGs are already fully qualified medical practitioners and their demotion to something akin to student level must challenge their ability to retain their professional identity. A strong professional identity as a medical doctor will assist through the process journey, but at the same time that identity is being eroded (Harris and Guillemin 2015). IMGs possess an occupational skill set if you like, and when that is questioned and tested, it represents a threat to occupational identity. While some IMGs may be undertaking some medical work, at the same time, their knowledge and skills are under examination. As they continue to work, their ability to work is being questioned. Therefore, IMGs may be able to utilise particular components of their occupational identity, by activation of parts of their "toolkit": "but it is the 'toolkit' itself that constitutes the entirety of one's occupational identity" (McDonald 2013, p. 242). The maintenance of identity for IMGs also involves the ability to finance the assessment journey they are required to undertake. For example, there is a financial cost to undertake examination assessment; application to enter a particular pathway attracts a fee as does appeals, cancellations and incomplete documentation.

## Strategies of Control: Fees

IMGs must be financially able to meet the costs associated with the practice of medicine in Australia. This requirement would immediately disadvantage some IMGs particularly those who are unemployed and those who, due to the circumstances they have come from, may be financially vulnerable. Compulsory fees represent another strategy to exclude and marginalise IMGs from the Australian medical profession. The system has an extensive array of fees with each of the speciality colleges having its own fee schedule. It is beyond the scope of this book to list them all; however, perhaps the most complex and expensive of all fee structures belongs to the RACS. This is not surprising as surgeons are at the top of the medical hierarchy. Currently, surgeons constitute the "most prestigious current professional of all (Susskind and Susskind 2015, p. 20). Table 1 is an example of fees required from IMGs by the RACS.

Unemployed IMGs must fund their fees from accumulated savings. This would be near impossible for those IMGs coming from poorer backgrounds or for those fleeing hostile unsafe countries, such as some refugee doctors. For those IMGs who can finance the fee requirements, their navigation through the process to registration may take several months to years. Harris and Guillemin (2015, p. 164) suggest that medically unemployed doctors: "are on the medical periphery and become part of the medical underground". Rita's story (2011, interview 4) is a case in point. In our interview, Rita mentioned that her husband (also an IMG) was driving a taxi while trying to study for his examinations. They both intended to practise medicine in Australia, but due to the extensive processes and fees required, Rita was forced to make a difficult decision. Rita abandoned her desire to practise medicine and found

**Table 1** RACS fees for IMGS (2016)

| | |
|---|---|
| Specialist assessment fee | 9504.00 |
| Supervision/oversight fee—onsite | 7620.00 |
| Supervision/oversight fee—remote | 21,750.00 |
| Document assessment fee—college endorsement for AoN | 1425.00 |
| Document assessment fee—AoN subsequent to specialist assessment | 1425.00 |
| IMG administration fee | 940.00 |
| Short-term specified training position application fee | 1140.00 |
| *Examinations* | |
| Clinical examination fee | 2170.00 |
| Fellowship examination fee | 7850.00 |
| Generic surgical science examination fee | 3780.00 |
| Speciality surgical science examination fee | 1890.00 |

employment as an assistant in a nursing home. Rita also managed to obtain some casual tutoring at the local university. There was sadness in her voice:

> We couldn't both do this it was too stressful on the family…my two little boys. I said you just study, no more taxis, and I will get a job. I wanted to maybe get into public health but they said I didn't have experience. It was a bit sad and friends and family they didn't understand…they said what are you doing! I had to see a Psychologist to help get through it (2011, interview 4).

Fees for profit have become a part of many aspects of modern society. Capitalism transformed and undermined traditional ideals and values. Profit became the primary motivation (Susskind and Susskind 2015). According to Blackshaw (2010, p. 162):

> One of the major reasons why the *status quo* is maintained (and capitalism flourishes) is that it readily incorporates from dissenting movements those aspects which dovetail with its *modus operandi*; while being always successful in resisting the remainder.

Hegemonic power enables the medical profession to demand payment of fees for the privilege of seeking approval to practise medicine. Ultimately, if an IMG is unable to pay the nominated fees, he or she cannot progress towards accreditation and registration. The following section reveals the voices of IMGs and their lived experience. The reader will gain an appreciation of what seems to be predominately a struggle with power; interpersonal power relations with the structural power of the system and the hegemonic power of the medical profession.

## Interpersonal Power: IMG Voices

In the context of interpersonal power, the following IMG experiences of the system are shared through the voices of the data set (focus group, individual interviews, the submissions to the 2012 Parliamentary Inquiry and 2016 Senate Committee Inquiry). The process journey for many IMGs can become a long-term struggle which seems to resemble a 'them' and 'us' battle. Unfortunately, some IMGs become defeated by the system and this position can be reflected in their inability to work in the capacity they desire, in their chosen profession, or the inability to work at all in their chosen profession, due to not meeting the requirements of the system. Subsequently, some IMGs experience adverse physical and or mental health issues. The story of Dr. D, a Canadian Assistant Professor of Family Medicine and past Head of Canada's largest obstetrics department, is a case in point.

Dr. D secured a lecturing position in the Australian National University's (ANU) medical school. However, on arrival and much to her dismay, she discovered that while she was considered highly qualified to teach Australian medical students, she was considered not sufficiently qualified (after seventeen years of clinical practice in Canada) to gain full registration to practise medicine in Australia. Dr. D was confronted with a lengthy and costly process journey. Dr. D wrote to the 2012 Parliamentary Inquiry Committee:

It isn't that any one event in itself is particularly shocking; it is the fact that the problems never seem to end, and just go on and on, to the point where you literally feel like you are losing your mind (2012, submission 111).

Dr. D was left feeling vulnerable and powerless. This eventually had an adverse impact on her mental health. Dr. D has been an outspoken representative for IMGs by her association with Australian Doctors Trained Overseas Association (ADTOA) and through her exposure in the media where she told of her struggles with the system. As a result, Dr. D told the 2012 inquiry that she has been contacted by over seventy overseas trained health professionals experiencing difficulties with the system. The majority were doctors, but she was also approached by dentists, nurses, pharmacists, physiotherapists and a vet. This indicates that other professional groups with qualifications from overseas also attract intense scrutiny from a system. My concern for the possible alienation of IMGs in this study from the system and perhaps from Australia itself due to their struggles convinces me to view IMGs as a community. This is an attempt to assign the IMG narratives through the stories they share, a central agency in the research with credibility and solidarity as a professional, political group.

## IMGs as a Professional Community

To further the agency of the IMG voice, I viewed them as a discrete community with professional solidarity. Following Anderson's idea of imagined community, IMGs can belong to their own community "because the members of even the smallest nation will never know most of their fellow-members, meet them, or even hear of them, yet in the minds of each lives the image of their communion" (Anderson 1983, p. 15). Further, Anderson believes that "communities are to be distinguished, not by their falsity/genuineness, but by the style in which they are imagined" (p. 6). In this sense, IMGs can view themselves as part of an IMG community while perhaps feeling as if they are somewhat excluded from the nation as outsiders. The power to identify as part of the nation is never equally distributed among a nation's members (Carter 2006). In fact, IMGs are represented by their own associations, such as the Australian Doctors Trained Overseas Association (ADTOA)[6], and there are other discipline-specific associations such as the Overseas Trained Specialist Anaesthetists Network (OTSAN). One FGP in this study made a comment that indicated a sense of community among IMGs; however, it also revealed vulnerability:

We network and support each other and stick together when we can. It's the blind leading the blind (Pascoe 2007).

A definition provided by Brint (2001, p. 8) views communities as: "aggregates of people who share common activities and/or beliefs and who are bound together *principally* by relations of affect, loyalty, common values, and/or personal concern". The

---

[6]Australian Doctors Trained Overseas Association (ADTOA) http://adtoa.org.au. Overseas Trained Specialist Anaesthetists Network (OSTAN) http://otsan.org/.

work of Patricia Hill Collins is particularly useful here. In her presidential address of 2010 to the American Sociological Association, she suggested the reframing of community as a political construct to advance new ways for investigating social inequalities. Community is either named as a political construct or implicated in political phenomena. Hill Collins (2010) advocates for rethinking intersecting systems of power and activities considered political for exploring how the construct of community works within power relations. The communal solidarity of the Australian trained doctors' community may be based on 'othering'. Following Bauman's ideas on liquid modern communities, Blackshaw (2010, p. 154) points out that the dark side of community solidarity operates by:

> Subjecting the least powerful social actors in communities…to a form of symbolic violence, which not only legitimizes the systems of meaning constructed in the interests of the powerful, but also maintains extant structures of social inequality.

In the eyes of the system, IMGs may, because of their lived experience, be labelled as not up to the standard of Australian trained doctors but IMGs can however constitute a community. The construct of community is an important tool in the organisation of power differentials between communities as well as a tool for use by people to challenge hierarchies. Underpinning the construct can be the idea of community as fundamental to group identification. If IMGs are viewed as a community, this implies a sense of solidarity.

According to Hill Collins (2010, p. 11): "the construct of community catalyses strong, deep feelings that can move people to action. Community is not simply a cognitive construct; it is infused with emotions and value-laden meanings". There is a social justice narrative entwined throughout the data which highlights the struggle, frustration and debilitation of some IMGs in Australia. As a result, the community construct is particularly relevant in this study. As Hill Collins (2010, p. 26) argues: "Community is a ubiquitous, versatile idea that can accommodate contradictory means and link thinking, feeling, and action in ways that make it especially useful for contemporary social justice initiatives". If IMGs wish to mobilise to become further empowered and take action, it seems that the best way to facilitate that would be via a community of IMGs rather than via individual IMGs.

Hence, in this study, IMGs can be positioned as the other in terms of their relationship with the system, but at the same time, as a discrete professional community. The other category brings with it an assumed deficit or inadequacy model because they are medical practitioners from overseas. The stumbling blocks constructed by the system are endemic. The underpinning rhetoric and justification for the extensive processes produced by the system always appears to be around maintaining the high standards that are expected in the Australian health system.

Surely the humans needing medical attention in Australia are not vastly different to humans needing medical attention elsewhere in the world. Dr. G (2012, submission 25) raised this with the Parliamentary Inquiry (2012) particularly in relation to the competent authority pathway which privileges doctors from New Zealand, the UK, Canada, USA and Ireland. This initiative seems to serve to divide IMGs into first-class IMGs and second-class IMGs and could be perceived as a racist initiative.

> The Competent Authority Pathway gave rise to a query of what['s] so special about doctors trained in the USA, UK, Canada and NZ? Isn't [it] that medical knowledge is a universal thing, regardless of language, colour, country status, the biochemical principles, human anatomical landmarks, mode of action of medications, types of bacteria and viruses, etc. are all the same wherever you are on Earth … Therefore there shouldn't be boundaries in categorising and assessing competency of an IMG regardless of country of origin (2012, submission 25).

The maintaining standards rhetoric seems a thinly veiled cover for the justification of such intense scrutiny and perhaps the potential for less scrutiny for IMGs from English-speaking countries considered 'more compatible' to Australian ways. Dr. A in his submission to the inquiry committee made clear his opinion of the maintaining standards rhetoric.

Dr. A argued that it is really about controlling competition:

> This has nothing to do with keeping standards; it is a closed shop mentality…don't expect these professional bodies to change their ways without considerable pressure. Which other profession is still in the extraordinarily privileged position to control national and global competition? (2012, submission 66).

There is difference however in the 'how' of medical practice, in the procedures, processes, protocols, rules and regulations from one country to another. The structure and agency relationship and associated discourses sit firmly entrenched within the boundaries of the system. The system communicates to IMGs via a deficit discourse which is a vehicle for power. In terms of this research relations of language and power are embodied in the discourses. These discourses and the associated practices of the many institutions which make up the system, overtly and covertly control IMGs.

## Discourse and Power

Initially, to provide a foundation on which to build an understanding of the IMG process and how it is experienced, it is necessary to explore the key concept of discourse and the complexity of power relations between the system and IMGs. For Foucault (1991), additional structures determine language use such as historically based combinations of various themes, concepts or problems. The language statements made around these structures become 'discursive formations'. A discourse becomes a collection of statements which are made by the same discursive formation. In this way, discourses frame understanding of identity and place in society and domination is constructed through discourses in particular social sites. Totalising discourses then refer to ways of thinking and acting which control and take over whole areas of human life (Foley 2000). For example, people's lives increasingly regulated by the practices and discourses of the professions (such as medicine) in that the population's health behaviours have become dominated by medical directive.

Rabinow (1984, p. 10) maintains that Foucault did not seek to isolate discourses from the surrounding social practices but rather his aim was to: "isolate techniques of power exactly in those places where this kind of analysis is rarely done". Foucault argued that it is more productive to explore the way power is constructed, than to identify the sources of domination and power. The construction of power in social institutions can be at the local or 'micro'-level and be subtle and undetected. This secret, unconscious aspect of discourses means that people can participate in their own subjugation by adopting the rules of a discourse or by accepting something that is socially constructed as 'truth'. In terms of this research, IMGs have no choice but to accept the discourses as they find themselves in a particularly vulnerable position. The socially constructed 'truth' of their situation they must engage with as 'truth' because it is a construction which has power over them and they are not familiar with it. If an IMG does not accept and follow the rules, he or she may be unable to get work as a doctor or at worst be deported from the country.

For example, an IMG who arrived in Australia in 2006 to take up work as a GP was deported. His anonymous story is one that highlights the amazing inflexibility of the system. The medical board advised the doctor in 2010 that despite being employed in a medical practice in an AON and ignoring the fact that he had completed, with results pending, the practice-based assessment (PBA) necessary for fellowship to the RACGP, he was to undergo the PESCI to renew his registration. Unfortunately, he failed and was advised that he was not fit to practise. Despite protests, requests and supporting documents, the medical board refused to renew his registration. On 1 July 2010, he was required to settle his affairs and return with his family to his country of origin. On 8 October 2010, he was informed that he had passed the PBA and was awarded fellowship to the RACGP in November 2010. Sadly, this successful outcome would not count. He wished to return to Australia with his family but was regrettably informed that he must begin the whole process again from the very beginning including supplying documents already supplied previously. This bureaucratic life-changing event has taken its toll on the doctor and his family:

> The income I have lost and the psychological challenge that my family and I had to go through is unquantifiable. If the medical board allowed me to renew my registration and allowed me to practice for another 4 months pending my PBA results then none of these would have happened (Anon 2012, submission 15).

The IMG/system relationship is characterised with systematic and sustained intervention. The discourses convey to IMGs that they constitute an inferior status. What is conveyed is essentially a deficit model. If an IMG is in constant struggle with the system and interaction is difficult and even demeaning, this will eventually impact on the IMG's concept of his or her self. Ideally, for Foucault (in Ball 1990, p. 2):

> Domination must be struggled with locally, dominant discourses must be countered by insurgent discourses: The only way to eliminate the fascism in our heads: is to explore and build upon the open qualities of human discourse, and thereby intervene in the way in which knowledge is produced in particular situations.

The self is made up of an individual's thoughts and feelings, and its construction is produced and influenced via interaction with others. A deficit ideology is at the core of the system/IMG interactions. The associated discourses establish, reflect and enforce deficit. Many IMGs in this study mention loss of confidence and loss of self-esteem due to their experiences with the system. In our interview, Colin shared an example from when he first arrived in Australia and attended an orientation session held in Brisbane:

> They went on and on about litigation, patients will sue you, you must be very careful. They made us feel like we don't know enough, and I got very nervous. For the first 3 months of work I lost my confidence even prescribing the most basic medication (2010, interview 2).

Similarly, a participant in Hawthorne et al.'s study explains his struggle with loss of confidence (2004, p. 45):

> Real life, real medicine starts here. Which I couldn't agree with. It came to a final situation (during a visit to a Melbourne hospital as part of an exam preparation course). They said, great, you have to forget about everything and accept what's going on. To start from zero. Then you pass exam and you start again. I couldn't get it. You know what I found? I started to lose my self-confidence. You realise that even if you pass exam and you lost confidence you are not a good doctor any more. And I tried to get something to preserve this confidence for me, professional confidence. The people in the bridging course we are trying to impress, and they are destroying our confidence completely.

Gorski (2010, p. 2) maintains the most devastating aspect of deficit thinking occurs: "when we mistake difference, particularly difference from ourselves, for deficit". In terms of this research, it is implied both overtly and covertly, sometimes subtly and sometimes blatantly, that IMGs may not meet the standards required for medical practice in Australia, simply because they are overseas trained. Harris (2009, p. 2) in her ethnographic study of overseas doctors in Victorian hospitals, also found that: "too often… the overseas doctors' difference is regarded, however subtly, in a negative way". The House of Representatives Inquiry and subsequent report (2012) noted that while many rural and remote communities have welcomed IMGs, they do not always receive the same level of support from the institutions and agencies that accredit and register them.

Moreover, the blatant exercise of power and intimidation by the system can be found in the fact that the report's forward also notes:

> Nearly one third of the IMGs who made submissions requested anonymity, citing fears that their chances of progressing through accreditation to registration would be compromised if it became known that they had commented publicly.

The fear of reprisal or penalty is not confined to IMGs. Interestingly, Knowles (2015) also makes mention in the Expert Advisory Group draft report on discrimination, bullying and sexual harassment for the Royal Australian College of Surgeons that some potential research participants (surgeons, trainees, consultants) were reluctant to take part in their research because of concerns for possible repercussions. Similarly, the 2016 Senate Inquiry experienced reluctance from some potential submitters towards speaking out.

If throughout the process journey an IMG receives negative messages and encounters negative interactions from the system to the extent that as a result, discourses culminate in fear, it may ultimately have adverse implications for his or her health and subsequent ability to practise medicine. In fact, in his submission to the 2012 inquiry, anaesthetist Dr. S, due to his first-hand experience of the "humiliating and depressing process" to get his professional qualification recognised in Australia, no longer recommends Australia as a professional destination (2012, submission 150). Minority group doctors generally can be vulnerable psychologically. From their 2013 National Mental Health Survey of Doctors and Medical Students, Beyond Blue concluded:

> minority groups such as overseas trained medical professionals, Indigenous doctors and students, and those working in rural and remote areas, where greater independence may be required with reduced access to support networks, have been identified as groups who may be particularly vulnerable to psychological distress (2013, p. 7).

Many experiences are based on seemingly ridiculous situations in which IMGs have found themselves due to the inflexible and almost bloody minded approach by the system, for example the case of Dr. T, an IMG from Kashmir. Dr. T was assessed, verified and granted provisional registration by the West Australian Medical Board on an annual basis and worked as a GP in an outer metropolitan area of Perth from 2004 to 2007. In 2008, new legislation required her to have her degree reverified because she was trained overseas. Dr. T was asked by the AMC to reapply for verification of her degree via the Educational Committee for Foreign Medical Graduates (ECFMG) which she did. The AMC and the ECFMG did not inform her of the progress, and when she eventually got a response to her repeated inquiries, she was told that they were waiting on the University of Kashmir. Dr. T contacted Kashmir herself and was told that due to an arson attack, student records prior to 1983 were destroyed. Dr. T offered to submit a true certified copy to the university, but this was declined. Apparently, the only option available to her was to post or personally present her original degree to the relevant university staff in Kashmir. Dr. T was not confident to let her degree out of her possession due to unstable and corrupt conditions in Kashmir, and described Kashmir as a war zone. In fact, the university's Vice-Chancellor was murdered in 1990. The Australian Government at the time had issued travel warnings, and Dr. T decided to heed the warnings:

> I felt it would be a significant danger to my life and safety…I am now not employed in any capacity (2012, submission 102).

Another example, which caused one interview participant to express anger and frustration in relation to the system's requirements, came to light in our interview. Tania was informed that she would have to resit the English assessment. Tania protested as she had already passed this assessment but was told there was no other option. Almost in tears (and in perfect English I might add), Tania said:

> This is crazy. I have done this and was successful. I have been in Australia for another two years since that, how could my English be worse? Why don't they stop disrupting our lives! (2011, interview 7).

Julian, another interview participant mentioned a particularly annoying situation where various bodies within the system refuse to share information. He was frustrated and amazed by the red tape in Australia but resigned to the fact that compliance is the only way through the system:

I needed some paperwork which I had to send for my initial registration. Now I needed it to be able to go to the exam with the RACGP and they actually refused to give, even a copy. I said "I need a copy of that paper." They said "We can't give you the original, you signed that, we keep that." I said "That's fine, I just need the copy. They only want the copy." It's a piece of paper I can only get from Europe again and they refused and they said "Look, we had a bad experience, blah, blah, blah, you could then copy it again and again and again, and it could go anywhere." And then I said "Look, if I get it from Europe, I could do the same as well. I could just copy it or change it or whatever." I really don't understand why they are so suspicious of OTDs generally. I think it is political…it's a kind of paranoia. I just have to get through it (2010, interview 1).

Dr. N after searching for a training position throughout Australia was finally offered an honorary position by a Melbourne hospital. His delight was subsequently dashed when, because he had not worked for one year, his registration and English language certificate had expired and as a result impacted his employment offer:

It is indeed very unfair to deprive me of the honorary position obtained with great difficulty because of the expiry of the validity of my English Language certificate by not renewing my specific registration. I believed once the English qualification was accepted by the Registration Board it remains valid as long as I am resident in Australia i.e. in an English speaking environment! (2012, submission 153).

The forward of the Parliamentary Inquiry's report (2012) further notes: "The Committee also had to contend with issues of a sensitive nature which had evidently resulted in high levels of angst and personal distress for some IMGs". For example, Dr. L wrote to the inquiry committee detailing his experiences of bullying in a NSW hospital and as a result:

I became very depressed and anxious. I could not sleep or eat and needed to take time off work for stress related reasons (2012, submission 118).

Similarly, Dr. D's endless struggle with the system's processes. Dr. D was advised that she had to obtain a fellowship with the College of General Practitioners before she could register as a GP; but she could not get a fellowship until she was registered stated:

I fell into a state of deep depression (2012, submission 111).

Dr. D obtained her medical qualifications in Canada, a competent authority pathway country. As a result, Dr. D should have gained greater recognition and easier access to registration in Australia. This was certainly not the case.

The 2016 Senate Community Affairs References Committee noted: "the large number of personal accounts from or on behalf of medical practitioners whose lives and careers had suffered" (2016, p. 39). For example, Dr. F told the Senate Committee (2016, p. 39) about the impact on himself and his family from having a vexatious complaint made against him and an investigation launched:

It changes you. It becomes all-consuming. You lose sleep. My wife and I spend hours beyond normal work hours trying to sort this out. It has affected our children with a combination of anxiety, depression and becoming more introverted. What should be a pleasant experience of helping people is now something you question every day: 'Why do I keep doing this? (Committee Hansard, 1 November 2016, p. 21).

The medical complaints process which is handled by AHPRA has also become a tool for bullying and harassment. Professor S discussed the additional impact on practitioners subjected to a vexatious complaint, sometimes leading to suicide:

> the significant unintended consequences of vexatious reporting, which causes practitioner illness, also causes severe financial hardship and, in a number of cases that we know about, has caused the suicide of very good doctors (Committee Hansard, November 2016, p. 13).

The Australian Medical Students' Association submission to the 2016 Senate Committee informed the inquiry that bullying begins during medical training. The Beyond Blue (2013) survey found that: "A fifth of medical students and almost a quarter of doctors reported thoughts of suicide over the preceding 12 months" (2016, submission 10).

IMG, Dr. L was subjected to appalling treatment by his supervisor. He informed the 2012 inquiry that he reported his experiences of bullying to three different organisations and was strongly encouraged to solve it privately and file a grievance rather than a bullying report. Dr. L stated that his supervisor told him:

> We will keep you like a dog on a leash. If you are a good puppy we will extend your leash, if not we will tighten it (2012, submission 118).

On another occasion when Dr. L questioned the low marks he had been given in a supervisory report, his supervisor informed him that the reason why was that:

> Top marks are reserved for the top 3% of best performers, and as you are overseas trained you cannot belong to this group (2012, submission 118).

Dr. L did report the bullying and was stunned to be advised that the same bullying supervisor he reported was nominated to investigate the allegations. He made the following analogy:

> I felt like a victim of rape asked to reconcile with the rapist (2012, submission 118).

Dr. L was told by the alleged bully that he had: "Dug a hole for himself". Eventually, he resigned his job, and as a result of his 'poor supervisory reports', the medical board imposed such strict conditions on Dr. L's registration that it made it almost impossible for him to find another position. During his efforts to find new employment, Dr. L was shocked to hear from a recruitment agency that his past supervisor had phoned the agency and instructed that Dr. L was not to be given any job. Baffled by this Dr. L stated:

> I have no idea why this man would go out of his way to track me down and sabotage my attempts to get a job (2012, submission 118).

Dr. L did find another position as a psychiatry trainee and at the time of writing was happy in his new location and felt lucky that his career was not totally ruined. However, the fact remains that as Dr. L concludes:

> My experiences at the hospital and its aftermath has inflicted serious damage to my career. I was deprived the opportunity to work in my profession, despite passing all required exams. I lost 11 months of my professional life and about $70,000.00 in income (2012, submission 118).

The 2012 examples of IMG narratives all tell of adverse experiences in their interactions with the system. Examples from within medicine generally given to the 2016 Senate Committee highlight the toxic culture of medicine. The fact that significant numbers of medical doctors and students contemplate suicide (as reported to the 2016 Senate Committee) is shocking. Moreover, the use of the AHPRA complaints process as a tool for bullying and harassment via vexatious complaints against colleagues is unacceptable. Another stark example is that of Dr. Da (2012) a highly qualified General Surgeon who was appointed to the position of General Surgeon at a rural South Australian hospital. It was made clear to Dr. Da that he was not welcome in surgical ranks. Dr. Da was given registration status with the[7] South Australian Medical Board of a non-vocationally trained general practitioner pending assessment by the AMC. Imagine arriving to begin your new job in an Australian hospital:

> I was met at the front door of the hospital by an Adelaide Professor of Surgery and informed that I was unwelcome in South Australia and should not consider travelling to Adelaide to partake in Surgical Departmental meetings, ward rounds etc., as general practitioners were not welcome at surgeons meetings (2012, submission 06).

Mechanisms were put in place to continually make it difficult if not impossible for Dr. Da to fulfil requirements. Post the Dr. Patel scandal of 2005 and the panic which ensued, registration requirements were tightened and supposedly streamlined such as the introduction of a centralised national registration process which was previously the responsibility of individual States. This initiative has been problematic and seems to still be inefficient. The following is Dr. Da's summary of his experiences and the subsequent tragic outcomes. This is an appalling story which shows a chain of events that led to the destruction of not only his career but his physical and mental well-being:

> I believe that as an IMG I have been: Used as a political pawn; invited and then made unwelcome, having burnt my bridges; rendered financially vulnerable and therefore manipulated; rendered professionally insecure with no mechanism to prove my worth; subjected to an unsympathetic employer prepared to take advantage of my predicament; dealt with by a nameless and faceless system impervious to my suffering; forced to negotiate with a devious College which continuously moved the goal posts and subjected to bullying.

> All the above resulted in my becoming initially hypertensive and then profoundly depressed and ultimately suicidal. I eventually sought professional help and have now withdrawn from many aspects of my former surgical practice. I will not return to my previous employment level (2012, submission 06).

The final irony was experienced by Dr. Da after years battling the system. A slightly inebriated senior surgeon announced to him: "Look, I like you, but we will never accept you as a surgeon in South Australia" (2012, submission 6). Dr. Da's submission not only highlights the inefficient, unreasonable and exclusionary practices by the system, but it also highlights the hierarchical structure of the medical system. Surgeons, for example, apparently outrank general medical practitioners. Dr.

---

[7]In 2006 COAG agreed to establish a single national registration scheme for health professionals. During 2009–2010 the National Registration and Accreditation Scheme (NRAS) was operationalised across Australia (Parliamentary Inquiry Report 2012, p. 9).

Da and Dr. L reveal the bullying culture within the medical profession. During our interview, Alex mentioned that he had been bullied by nurses; perhaps, nursing staff are positioned above IMGs in the medical hierarchy:

> The nurses were bullies, they said I was rude to them and they talked about 'certain' doctors in front of me like I was not present. (I knew they were talking about me)...he's this and he's that and they laughed. I was very uncomfortable. In my culture we don't say please and thank you all the time...does that mean I'm rude? I was glad to leave that hospital and them (2012, interview 10).

There are many stories like these in the data, many casualties from the maze that is the process journey for IMGs. It seems that on the one hand while Australia relies on IMGs, on the other hand Australia does everything it can to make it difficult for IMGs, why is this the case? Power relations are at play here; it is the immense hegemonic power of the system which creates and maintains these conditions. In Australia: "Medicine dominates the health division of labour economically, politically, socially and intellectually"(Willis 1989, p. 2). Dr. G gave his opinion to the 2012 Parliamentary Inquiry Committee:

> It is my opinion that the present and future shortage of doctors in Australia is an artificially maintained phenomenon, which is based on pecuniary considerations of incumbents. It is created by the legislatively protected monopoly of the medical market place. This monopoly of local graduates is enforced by the existing legislation and by the modus operandi of the registering authorities (2012, submission 31, p. 2).

The data clearly indicates that the IMG experience in Australia is impacted by a group of interconnected systems of oppression that together form a single, historically created system with systemic power, that of the Australian health system. Intersectionality is a particularly useful framework here as it not only seeks to critique the work of power, but by exploring why the social world is structured the way it is, the work of power is also confronted. Understanding of how power is operationalised, and its impact has the potential for challenge and ultimately transformation (Hill Collins 2000). The following examples focus on how some IMGs view and experience the hegemonic power operationalised through the subjugation of IMGs as a source of cheap labour.

According to Dr. G, the rates of pay for IMGs generally are maintained at the minimum. Is this a deliberate strategy to indeed treat IMGs as a source of cheap labour? Even more concerning, Dr. G mentioned that an IMG who questions employment conditions can be easily dismissed based on alleged poor performance.

> As a general rule OTDs are paid minimal allowed rates and, if this Doctor would ask for his or her pay to be on par with the accepted rates, or request a raise promised at the time of the beginning of the employment, the shortcomings of his/her care provision would be found and this OTD would be quietly dismissed (2012, submission 31 p. 2).

Another example was offered by Surgeon Dr. Da whose account not only reveals a cheap labour situation but also one of dishonesty on the part of a hospital to save money:

The X Hospital management informed me that my registration status was immaterial to them as I would work exclusively as a general surgeon and also perform all the emergency orthopaedic surgery. I was on call twenty four out of every twenty eight days. My name did not however appear on the duty roster for twelve of those twenty four nights, thereby saving the hospital the standby allowance for 50% of my after hours' work…The Adelaide surgeons received eleven times the standby allowance for performing the same work as I did (2012, submission 06).

A participant in Hawthorne et al.'s study (2004, p. 43) was only able to secure a more equitable wage after intervention from the AMA on his behalf:

When I first came, I came on a salary so it did not matter that much how much I see patients at all. But after I knew that was very little – they gave me $800 per week – which I was very happy to take as I didn't know much because I wasn't working before, and I could still pay tax out of that $800, rent and everything. Then another doctor I met said to ask the AMA. So I did ask the AMA, and they said no, that's very minimal and we can negotiate for you if you want. So they negotiated for me and they put my salary up to $1200 at first, then $1500.

Hawthorne et al. (2004, pp. 40–41) found four key themes (including appropriate remuneration) in relation to colleagues' attitudes repeatedly occurred in their study; these were:

1. Peer wariness or distrust of medical outsiders (in some cases perceived as downright hostility);
2. Lack of respect for the overseas trained doctor's skills, including his/her ability to deal with a range of cases without vetting;
3. Reluctance of other doctors to refer on an adequate flow of patients (despite OTDs recognition of the commitment made by many Australian colleagues to building up patient lists); and
4. Unwillingness to allocate the OTD sufficient remuneration.

Do IMGs appeal against unfair conditions? Appeals are expensive and often unsuccessful. Dr. G made comment as to the impossibility of fair appeal for IMGs seeking to report workplaces or to appeal decisions made by medical bodies within the system. In fact, Dr. G believed that to appeal was a waste of time and money due to power, control and legal protection:

The registering bodies or a body now, are not answerable to anyone with the political clout to change their decisions. The hypothetical possibility of going to the Administrative Appeals Tribunal or Human Rights Commission is useless because these organisations, having tackled Medical Boards before, learned the awesome power of the legal protection these registering bodies enjoy. Who would wish to squander limited resources on a hopeless quest? In the end OTDs are left unprotected (2012, submission 31).

Dr. D was optimistic enough to undertake the appeals process and mentioned that the RACGP appeals guidelines state that an answer would be forthcoming within fourteen working days. It was actually nine months before Dr. D received communication from the college. The letter stated that a reconsideration of a decision was declined, but she was welcome to apply for the second stage of appeal. Interestingly, Dr. D received another letter to say that her file had been reviewed and there was no original application form; therefore, she had no basis for appeal. The letter stated:

"On consideration of the events it is clear that there was no valid application before the RACGP. There is therefore no decision which might attract the appeals process." Dr. D was mystified: "It is difficult to understand how the board could have made a decision on my application if I had never filed an application" (2012, submission 111).

Dr. BJ has become an Australian citizen and has lived in Australia for over twenty years. Despite also completing a PhD in endocrinology through the University of Sydney and the Royal Prince Alfred Hospital, he has been seeking registration since 1993. Due to the obvious errors associated with his clinical examination feedback letter with no result recorded, Dr. BJ sought legal advice:

I spent more than $15,000 for legal advice from two barristers. They advised me to give up, as it would cost a fortune. A solicitor from the college also advised me to do so (2012, submission 26).

Through the lived experiences of IMGs presented here, a complex process journey is revealed. Of course, some IMGs do not experience difficulties with their process journey. In terms of this study, one interview participant (Barry) did not have any negative comments to make. For example, Barry was very pleased with his employment situation:

At our practice we take every day from 12.00–2.00 pm to eat our lunch together and discuss cases. Everybody is helpful and I like my work. I feel welcome and I know that there is a lot of red tape to get through here but that is a good necessary thing for the patients (2011, interview 6).

Hawtorne et al.'s study (2004, p. 32) found: "Encouragingly, 40 per cent of respondents reported being very satisfied with the nature of their GP work, compared to 56% who were only reasonably satisfied and 4% who were dissatisfied". The following are examples of positive interview responses:

Family and friends in this area, lifestyle, the local circumstances are from a work perspective excellent. I work in a good practice, it's a relatively young group of GPs, there are registrars here whose education is interesting, evidence-based medicine, so it's very stimulating. I'm able to work and for the family it's a very pleasant environment to live. Not too far away from family and friends so it's the best of both worlds, I would say (p. 34).

I liked it and I love it too now. I come from a relatively poor country not well organised, so it is still all amazing for me. Organised, well planned in advance, ongoing education. It is unreal for us. You can get any information, any support, anything you need in terms of your medical problems - you can do anything. I was pleasantly surprised and I'm enjoying it (p. 35).

"In general British-origin doctors reported the most streamlined transitions. Doctors from Asia, Africa and the Middle East were 3 times more likely to be only reasonably satisfied or to be actively dissatisfied" (Hawthorne et al. 2004, pp. 34–37). Unfortunately, below is the negative account of a participant from Hawthorn et al.'s study (2004, pp. 38–39) detailing racism towards his son at school culminating in the family's relocation from a rural area to Melbourne:

We have suffered a lot. We are heroes to do all this. In this countryside there's one high school and my son is dark colour and this (town) is a very Australian closed society, there's no multiculturalism, not people from any other nations. There's just a few recent Asians because of the Australians going to marry some who are coming here. They also have two takeaways owned by Asian people, but other than that there's no other nationalities in that town. Very big difficulty with my son, going to that school all these years, every day Saddam Hussein always on the news, you are from Iraq, go back to your bloody country. He had all that kind of racism, made me transfer him to three high schools (including one an hour's drive away)… My kids are now going to Melbourne so I have to move to Melbourne to be at least with my kids, be paid better, not be (suffering) racism.

The structure of the system and its systemic power, and the hegemonic power of the Australian medical profession have a far-reaching impact on IMGs, their careers, their families and their well-being. For some IMGs, constant struggle with the system has defeated them and they experience undermined self-confidence and adverse mental health issues. Kemper (2011, p. 236) argues that: "happiness indicates sufficient status, sadness indicates irremediably insufficient status, anger indicates status withdrawn or withheld undeservedly, and fear indicates the threat of power from other. Anticipatory emotions then arise such as optimism/pessimism or confidence/lack of confidence". An analysis of the power differential and the positioning of IMGs has been revealed. It is clear that the structural power of the system has been created and continues to be maintained, with one of its objectives being: to tightly control the accreditation and registration of IMGs. Via a deficit discourse, the qualifications of IMGs are rigorously questioned, assessed and tested. The hegemonic power of the Australian medical profession has enabled the concept of deficit to be firmly embedded in the system and its processes. The interpersonal power of IMGs is severely compromised as they are unable to successfully hold the system to account. IMGs are essentially dependent on the system to grant them the accreditation and registration that is mandatory for them to practise their profession. Relations of power and associated discourses have been explored through the structural, hegemonic and interpersonal power domains to enable insight into how IMGs are positioned within Australia's medical culture.

This chapter explains the concept of medical dominance and explores how this has developed and changed over time. In addition, a major task of this book, which is to explore why medical dominance is created, mobilised and maintained, is offered. The evolvement of a toxic culture within Australian medicine is also revealed, constituting a culture of bullying and an uncompetitive, self-interest agenda.

# References

Anderson, B. (1983). *Imagined communities: Reflections on the origin and spread of nationalism.* London: Verso.

Australian College of Rural and Remote Medicine. (2016). Viewed September 12, 2016, http://www.acrm.org.au/.

Australian Government Department of Immigration and Border Protection. (2016). *Australian Government*, viewed October 5, 2016, https://www.border.gov.au.

Australian Health Practitioner Regulation Agency. (2016). Viewed August 24, 2016, http://www.ahpra.gov.au.

Australian Institute of Health and Welfare. (2015). *Who are medical practitioners*, viewed September 8, 2016, www.aihw.gov.au/workforce/medical/who.

Australian Medical Council. (2016). Viewed 10 June 2016, www.amc.org.au/assessent/clinical-exam.

Ball, S. (1990). *Foucault and education*. London: Routledge.

Belcher, H. (2014). Power, politics, and health care. In J. Germov (Ed.), *Second opinion: An introduction to health sociology* (pp. 359–387). VIC: Oxford University Press.

Betta, M. (2016). *Ethicmentality—Ethics in capitalist economy, business, and society*. Springer, viewed May 7, 2017, https://doi.org/10.1007/978-94-017-7590-8, http://www.springer.com/series/6077.

Beyond Blue. (2013). *National mental health survey of doctors and medical students*. viewed 12 October 2015, www.beyondblue.org.au.

Blackshaw, T. (2010). *Key concepts in community studies*. London: Sage Key concepts series, Sage Publications.

Bonditti, P., Bigo, D., & Gros, F. (Eds.) (2017). *Foucault and the modern international: Silences and legacies for the study of world politics*. Springer Palgrave Macmillan.

Brint, S. (2001). Gemeinschaft revisited: A critique and reconstruction of the community concept. *Sociological Theory, 19*(1), 2–23, viewed February 27, 2014, via ProQuest Central (Flinders university SA).

Carter, D. (2006). *Dispossession, dreams & diversity: Issues in Australian studies*. Frenchs Forest, NSW: Pearson Education Australia.

Cohen, E. (2017). Dare to care: Between Stiegler's mystagogy and Foucault's aesthetics of existence. *Boundary 2, 44*(1), 150–166, viewed May 6, 2017, https://doi.org/10.1215/01903659-3725917.

Commonwealth Department of Health. (2016). *DoctorConnect*, Australian Government, viewed August 24, 2016, www.doctorconnect.gov.au.

Crampton, J. W., & Elden, S. (2016). *Space, knowledge and power: Foucault and geography*. London: Routledge Taylor and Francis Group.

Dawes, S. (2016). Foucault-phobia and the problem with the critique of neoliberal ideology: A response to Downey et al. *Media, Culture and Society, 38*(2), 284–293, viewed May 7, 2017, https://doi.org/10.1177/0163443715610922, mcs.sagepub.com.

Depew, J. F. (2016). Foucault among the stoics: Oikeiosis and counter-conduct. *Foucault Studies, 21*, 22–51, viewed May 5, 2017, https://rauli.cbs.dk/index.php/foucault-studies/index.

Educational Commission for Foreign Medical Graduates. (2016). Viewed November 2, 2016, http://www.ecfmg.org.

Foley, G. (Ed.). (2000). *Understanding adult education and training* (2nd ed.). Crows Nest: Allen & Unwin.

Foucault, M. (1991). Governmentality. In G. Burchell, C. Gordon, & P. Miller (Eds.), *The Foucault effect: studies in governmentality* (pp. 87–104). Hertfordshire: Harvester Wheatsheaf.

Gariepy, K. D. (2016). *Power, discourse, ethics: A policy study of Academic Freedom*. Sense Publishers, Rotterdam, The Netherlands, viewed May 5, 2017, https://www.sensepublishers.com.

Germov, J. (2005). Managerialism in the Australian public health sector: Towards the hyper-rationalisation of professional bureaucracies. *Sociology of Health & Illness, 27*(6), 738–758.

Germov, (Ed.). (2014). *Second opinion* (5th ed.). South Melbourne, Australia: Oxford University Press.

Gordon, C. (Ed.). (1980). *Power/knowledge: Selected interviews and other writings 1972–1977 Michel Foucault*. Sussex: Harvester press.

Gorski, P. C. (2010). *Unlearning deficit ideology and the scornful gaze: Thoughts on authenticating the class discourse in education*. Fairfax: George Mason University.

Hampton, T. (2016). *What is a colony before colonialism? Humanist and antihumanist concepts of governmentality from Foucault to Montaigne*, 5, Palgrave Macmillan, 978-3-319-32276-6 (eBook).

Hanson, C., & Ogunade, A. (2016). Caught up in power: Exploring discursive frictions in Community Research. *Gateways: International Journal of Community Research and Engagement, 9*(1),

41–57, viewed May 7, 2017, https://doi.org/10.5130/1jcre.v911.4729, https://epress.lib-uts.edu.au/journals/index.php/1jcre/index.

Harris, A. (2009). *Overseas doctors in Australian hospitals: An ethnographic study of how degrees of difference are negotiated in medical practice*. PhD thesis, University of Melbourne.

Harris, A. (2011). Doctors from overseas are being wasted. *The Age, Opinion and Society*, April 7, 2011.

Harris, A., & Guillemin, M. (2015). Notes on the medical underground: Migrant doctors at the margins. *Health Sociology Review, 24*(2), 163–174, viewed March 21, 2016, http://dx.doi.org/10.1080/14461242.2014.999403.

Hawthorne, L., Birrell, B., & Young, D. (2004). *The Retention of Overseas Trained Doctors in General Practice in Regional Victoria*. pp. 1–100.

Hill Collins, P. (2000). *Black feminist thought: Knowledge consciousness, and the politics of empowerment* (2nd ed.). New York: Routledge.

Hill Collins, P. (2010). The new politics of community. *American Sociological Review, 75*(1), 7–30, viewed September 6, 2012, https://doi.org/10.1177/0003122410363293, via Sage (dowloaded from asr.sagepub.com at Adelaide theological library) http://asr.sagepub.com.

Hodges, B. D., Martimianakis, M. A., McNaughton, N., & Whitehead, C. (2014). Medical Education…Meet Michel Foucault. *Medical Education, 48,* 563–571. https://doi.org/10.1111/medu.12411.

House of Representatives Standing Committee on Health and Ageing. (2012). *Lost in the Labyrinth: Report on the inquiry into registration processes and support for overseas trained doctors*. Canberra: The Parliament of the Commonwealth of Australia.

Hyland, T. (2011). Foreign doctors' obstacle course 'a disgrace'. *The Age*, November 20.

Iredale, (2009). Luring overseas trained doctors to Australia: Issues of training, regulating and trading. *International Migration, 47*(4), 31–64.

Keleher, H. (2016). The medical profession in Australia. In E. Willis, L. Reynolds, & H. Keleher (Eds.), *Understanding the Australian health care system* (3rd ed., pp. 395–408). Chatswood, NSW: Elsevier.

Kemper, T. D. (2011). *Status, power and ritual interaction: A relational reading of Durkheim, Goffman and Collins*. Surrey, England: Ashgate publishing.

Knowles, R. (2015). *Expert Advisory Group draft report on discrimination, bullying and sexual harassment*. Royal Australasian College of Surgeons. http://www.surgeons.org/media/22045685/eag-report-to-racs-draft-08-sept-2015.pdf.

Legg, S. (2016). Subject to truth: Before and after governmentality in Foucault's 1970s. *Environment and Planning D: Society and Space, 34*(5), 858–876, viewed May 6, 2017, https://doi.org/10.1177/0263775816633474, epd.sagepub.com.

Lorenzini, D. (2016). From counter-conduct to critical attitude: Michel Foucault and the art of not being Governed quite so much. *Foucault Studies, 21*, 7–21, viewed May 7, 2017, https://rauli.cbs.dk/index.php/foucault-studies/index.

McCall, C. (2016). Rituals of conduct and counter-conduct. *Foucault Studies, 21*, 52–79, viewed May 7, 2017, https://rauli.cbs.dk/index.php/foucault-studies/index.

McDonald, S. (Ed.). (2013). *Networks, work and inequality* (Vol. 24), Research in the sociology of work, Emerald Group Publishing, UK.

Medical Board of Australia. (2016). Australian Government, viewed August 30, 2016, http://www.medicalboard.gov.au.

Nguyen, K. H. (2017). *Rhetoric in Neoliberalism*. In K. H. Nguyen (Ed.), Palgrave Macmillan, Switzerland, viewed May 6, 2017, https://doi.org/10.1007/978-3-319-39850.1, http://books.google.com.au/.

Nica, E. (2017). Foucault on managerial governmentality and biopolitical neoliberalism. *Journal of Self Governance and Management Economics, 5*(1), 80–86.

Ninnis, D. (2016). Foucault and the madness of classifying our madness. *Foucault Studies, 21*, 117–137, viewed May 7, 2017, https://rauli.cbs.dk/index.php/foucault-studies/index.

Pascoe, V. A. (2007). *International medical graduates—Focus group*. X Division of General Practice.

Peters, M. A. (2017). *Education in a post-truth world: Educational philosophy and theory*. p. 4, viewed May 12, 2017, https://doi.org/10.1080/00131857.2016.1264114.

Powell, J. L. (2015). Foucault, power and culture. *International Journal of Humanities and Cultural Studies, 1*(4), 401–419, viewed May 8, 2017, http://ijhcschiefeditor.wix.com/ijhcs.

Rabinow, P. (Ed.). (1984). *The Foucault reader: An introduction to Foucault's thought, with major new unpublished material*. London, England: Penguin books.

Raffnsoe, S., Gudmand-Hoyer, M., & Thaning, M. S. (2016). Foucault's dispositive: The perspilacity of dispositive analytics in organisational research. *Organization, 23*(2), 272–298, viewed May 6, 2017, https://doi.org/10.1177/1350508414549885, http://www.org.sagepub.com.

Rural Health Workforce Australia. (2016). Viewed September 5, 2016, http://www.rhwa.org.au/International-Recruitment-Strategy.

Schroder, S., & Thompson, C. (2015). A matter of exposition: Examination and education. *Ethics and Education, 10*(2), 152–162, viewed September 12, 2016, www.tandonline.com/doi/abs/10.1080/17449642.2015.1039273.

Susskind, R., & Susskind, D. (2015). *The future of the professions: How technology will transform the work of human experts*. New York: Oxford University Press.

Tazzioli, M. (2016). Revisiting the omnes et singulatim bond: The production of irregular conducts and the Biopolitics of the Governed. *Foucault Studies, 21*, 98–116, viewed May 7, 2017, https://rauli.cbs.dk/index.php/foucault-studies/index.

The Senate Community Affairs Committee. (2016). *Medical complaints process in Australia, Report*. Commonwealth of Australia. Viewed 12 January 2017, https://www.aph.gov.au/Parliamentary_Business/Committees/Senate/Community_Affairs/MedicalComplaints45/Report.

Turner, B. S. (1995). *Medical power and social knowledge* (2nd ed.). London: Sage Publications.

Twohig, J. (2016). The complementary and alternative health care system in Australia. In E. Willis, L. Reynolds, & H. Keleher (Eds.), *Understanding the Australian health care system* (pp. 207–224). Chatswood: Elsevier.

Villadsen, K. (2016). Michael Foucault and the forces of civil society. *Theory, Culture and Society, 33*(3), 3–26, viewed September 17, 2016 (Downloaded from tcs.safepub.com at Flinders University South Australia).

Wang, D. (2017). *Foucault and the smart city*. Paper presented to Design for Next: 12th EAD Conference, Sapienza University of Rome, April 12–24, 2017, http://eprints.lancs.ac.uk?85521/1/DfN-full-paper-DW.

Willis, E. (1989). *Medical dominance: The division of labour in Australian health care* (Revised Edn.), North Sydney: Allen & Unwin.

Willis, E. (2006). Introduction: Taking stock of medical dominance. *Health Sociology Review, 15*(5), 421–431.

World Directory of Medical Schools. (2016). Viewed September 25, 2016, http://www.wdoms.org/.

Zamora, D. (2016). Introduction: Foucault, the left, and the 1980s. In D. Zamora & M. C. Behrent (Eds.), *Foucault and Neoliberalism*.

# Medical Dominance and the Creation of Toxic Culture

A profession attains and maintains its position by virtue of the protection and patronage of some strategic elite segment of society which has been persuaded that there is some special value in its work. Its position is thus secured by the political and economic influence of the elite which sponsors it-an influence that drives competing occupations out of the same area of work, that discourages others by virtue of the competitive advantages conferred on the chosen occupation and that requires still others to be subordinated to the profession. (Freidson 1970b, pp. 72–73)

Collectively, we must change the often toxic culture of medicine into a culture that promotes a nurturing and supportive approach to teaching and supervision. The goal should be to develop medical practices that facilitate well-being and quality of life, where sustainable medical careers can develop and better serve the community. (Ward and Outram 2016, p. 112)

The role of chapter five is to transport the reader to the application of power. The origin of power, as it is manifested in the medical profession, is explored and the concept of medical dominance is explained and unpacked. Willis' (1989) noteworthy and influential work in the area of medical dominance explores the division of labour in the health system particularly the influence of the state. Dominance is viewed as control over esoteric knowledge, or medical knowledge known only to the medical profession, which is maintained by the interface between the economy and the State. For Willis (1989), there are three levels of medical dominance: firstly over medicine's work, secondly over the work of other health practitioners and thirdly over society. Willis (1989, p. 8) argues that: "dominance at each level is represented by the concepts of autonomy, authority and medical sovereignty". It is important to note that while medical dominance prevails in Australia at the time of writing, it has been challenged and as a result, changes shape to meet these challenges. The profession has been challenged on various levels from the increasingly aware Internet patient to the increased public interest in alternate and complementary therapies.

The gap in the literature addressed by this book is demonstrated in the questioning of how and why IMGs are placed within medical dominance and crucially to explore why medical dominance positions and continues to position IMGs as an underclass

© Springer Nature Singapore Pte Ltd. 2019
V. A. Pascoe, *Australia's Toxic Medical Culture*,
https://doi.org/10.1007/978-981-13-2426-0_5

within an elite profession. The analysis of medical dominance must look at how it has come about and how it is reproduced over time. The 'how' is an important part of analysis, but equally important I believe, is the 'why'. An exploration of the 'why' is a fundamental part in the move towards understanding the position of IMGs in Australia. For Willis (1989, p. 3) "occupational ideology legitimating autonomy" sets the terms for the health division of labour. Medicine has control over other health professions such as pharmacy, optometry and dentistry. This is an indirect control, however, that is operationalised through strategies such as setting the legal boundaries of these occupations and a medical presence on their registration boards. Subsequently, ongoing influence retains control of processes. Moreover, the medical profession has the power to exclude various health occupations by denying them official legitimacy and assigning them an 'alternate' status. How does the Australian public feel about this domination when it is clear that there is growing interest in complementary and alternate health therapies?

## What is Expected from the Medical Profession?

The Australian public have, in good faith, entrusted the provision of appropriate medical services to the government and the medical profession. The Australian public should surely expect the profession to behave ethically and in the public's best interests. Medical practitioners are subject to a code of ethics. The Geneva Declaration or the Hippocratic Oath and the AMA[1] outline core elements to ethical practice for doctors. These include respect patient confidentiality, do not harm or abuse patients, do not undertake work beyond level of competence and provide equal treatment of patients (Keleher 2016). Perhaps the Australian public assume that an unspoken deal or bargain has been struck with the medical profession in return for the public's trust and respect. After analysis of the professions and a study of the literature, Susskind and Susskind (2015, p. 22) suggest the following social contract:

> In acknowledgement of and in return for their expertise, experience, and judgement, which they are expected to apply in delivering affordable, accessible, up-to-date, reassuring, and reliable services, and on the understanding that they will curate and update their knowledge and methods, train their members, set and enforce standards for the quality of their work and that they will only admit appropriately qualified individuals into their ranks, and that they will always act honestly, in good faith, putting the interests of clients ahead of their own, we (society) place our trust in the professions in granting them exclusivity over a wide range of socially significant services and activities, by paying them a fair wage, by conferring upon them independence, autonomy, rights of self-determination, and by according them respect and status.

Freidson (1970a) deemed medicine as the archetype profession which should, as all professions, adopt the provision of strong ethical service. Conversely, the preceding IMG narratives indicate that many doctors from overseas have encountered

[1] The full Geneva Declaration: ama.com.au/media/ama-adopts-wma-declaration-geneva, The AMA Code of Ethics: atama.com.au/position-statement/ama-code-ethics-2004-editorially-revised-2006.

particularly unethical behaviours and practices at the hands of the medical profession. Yet, the profession is gifted with not only the trust of the general public but also the State. According to Willis et al. (2016, p. 6) in their discussion of the Australian health system and in this case particularly medicine:

> Trust is given to professionals by the State and the patient because it is assumed that they work in the interest of their patients with a high level of skill underpinned by a high level of education. This gives the profession considerable esteem in the eyes of patients.

It would appear that the proposed social contract above expects the system to assess the qualifications and skills of IMGs seeking to practise medicine in Australia. It is of course necessary to ensure that the standard of health care in Australia is maintained, therefore medical doctors with qualifications from overseas, wishing to practise medicine in Australia should be assessed, but how much assessment is adequate and for how long? Perhaps in the spirit of maintaining high standards IMGs are administered an assessment overdose. I argue that there is far more at stake here than assessment to ensure the high standards of Australia's healthcare system are maintained. Rather, while ensuring overseas medical qualifications meet Australian health standards is a necessary and noble exercise, this is not entirely the reason. The intense scrutiny and assessment of IMGs is also very much driven by jealousy, conflict of interests, commercial gains and market share. The data indicates that IMGs are often not afforded full admission to the medical profession even after years of exemplary practice in Australia. One IMG informed the 2012 Parliamentary Inquiry Committee: "I have been in this country for twenty years, I am an Australian citizen but I will always be overseas trained" (2012, submission 26). After years of practice in this country, this doctor does not feel a 'genuine' part of the Australian medical profession. It is helpful to begin with an exploration of how the Australian medical profession managed to obtain the power it currently enjoys and waves over the heads of IMGs, other health professionals and the general public. An historical lens will provide the reader with an appreciation of the rise of the medical profession. The focus concern then is to trace how the Australian medical practitioner has obtained a powerful elite status and what has influenced and directed this over time. As Bacchi (2009, p. 43) suggests: "In Genealogy, attention is directed to the power relations that allowed and allow particular problem representations to emerge and gain status". The medical profession in Australia, despite changing demands, manages to retain its elite status. Is this status earned or ascribed?

## The Rise of the Medical Profession

The 1870s marked a change in the professional status of doctors. At the time, there were advances in medical science which initiated change in medical practice in the colony. Doctors were increasingly able to present themselves above alternate prac-titioner competitors. These practitioners included "chemists, dentists, herbalists and medical clairvoyants. Under the Medical Practitioners Act of 1862, these practitioners could not adopt formal titles but were free to treat the sick for a fee" (Pensabene 1980, p. 5). In contemporary, Australia not only do medical doctors present themselves above alternate and complimentary health practitioners but they also have the power to contain them to the healthcare margins (Twohig 2016).

Pharmacists were in direct competition with registered doctors not only because of their knowledge of diseases and drugs but also because, according to Pensabene (1980, p. 9) they offered 'shop front' medical care:

> The chemist was the first source of medical care for the majority of individuals…the chemist was located close to the main sources of public transport and accessible to most people. In addition…large chemists provided mail ordering services, posting medicines to distant patients. The patient had only to consult the daily newspapers to ascertain the types of treatment obtainable through the mail.

Some of the medications sold by chemists made unbelievable curative claims and contained dangerous concoctions. For example, medicines advertised to cure impure blood-related diseases such as cancer and 'nervous trouble' usually contained a substantial amount of gin. The medicine with the comforting name of 'Mrs Winslow's Soothing Syrup' was made to treat teething children and contained among other ingredients, morphine. A New South Wales Department of Health report found: "most patent medicines contained high quantities of opium, morphine or chloroform". Unregistered practitioners were also readily consulted by the public (Lewis 2014). This range of practitioners constituted a curious group and included, as identified by the 1881 Victorian census (Pensabene 1980, p. 7): "aurists and oculists, homeopaths, hydropathists, herbalists, medical galvanists, medical botanists, medical mesmerists, medical clairvoyants and psychopathists". Variations of these alternate practices are currently operating in Australia, such as medical herbalists and practitioners of homeopathy.

As in the 1800s, many Australians prefer to consult a chemist before seeking out the services of a medical practitioner. Consumers expect pharmacies to carry a stock of complementary products and: "75% of Australians have used them" (Carter 2016, p. 380). The Australian medical profession, however, does not share the enthusiasm and actively works to discredit complementary and alternative medicine (CAM). Twohig (2016, p. 210) maintains: "Opposition still exists in sections of the medical profession and is supported by the often-vitriolic attacks directed towards CAM". Many consider CAM pseudo-science, and an example of opposition was demonstrated by the Friends of Science in Medicine's unsuccessful campaign to stop universities offering CAM courses (Brosnan 2015). The practice of CAM tends to be absent in government policies, and many practitioners are denied national registration (Twohig 2016).

However, according to the Australian Institute of Health and Welfare (AIHW) complementary and alternative health services have been marginally incorporated into the health system. For example, acupuncture when practised by a medical practitioner can be eligible for a Medicare rebate. Acupuncture rebates such as these constituted:

A total of 0.6 million claims… in 2004–05, attracting benefits paid of $20.0 million. Some private health ancillary insurance covers some of these services, such as those provided by naturopaths, osteopaths, chiropractors and acupuncturists. In the quarter ending September 2005, there were benefits paid for approximately 1.8 million chiropractic services, 0.5 million natural therapy services, 0.3 million acupuncture/acupressure services and 51,000 osteopathic services. (Australian Institute of Health and Welfare 2006, p. 395)

Australian Bureau of Statistics (ABS) figures show that while there has been a consistent and considerable rise in the patronage of CAM, it still occupies a marginalised health space: "People consulting a CAM professional increased by 51% in the 10 years to 2005. Almost 750,000 people had visited a CAM practitioner in a two week period and the number of people working as CAM professionals rose from 4800 to 8600 in the 10 years to 2006" (Australian Bureau of Statistics 2008; Burnet 1939). There is still a xenophobic suspicion among the orthodox Australian medical profession around 'other' practitioners and this was also evident in the 1800s. Pensabene (1980, p. 17) points out that prior to 1970 no doctor with Chinese qualifications was entitled to registration as a legally qualified practitioner. The case of Doctor Yee, highly proficient in acupuncture, is an example of early xenophobia. Doctor Yee met all requirements of the Medical Act, and his qualifications were recognised by the Chinese government, he was the first Chinese doctor to apply for registration. European mistrust of Chinese medicine, however, prevented Yee from being registered. The medical board sought the opinion of the British Magistrate Legation in Peking, who advised that Doctor Yee had: "no knowledge of medicine or surgery other than that gained from Chinese works which are fearfully incorrect as might be expected in the case of people who protest against anatomy as mutilation". Pensabene (1980, p. 17) also notes that there was no objection, however, to: "Yee and other Chinese doctors treating patients of their own nationality". Many Australians now embrace acupuncture as a treatment and there are many Australians who practise as acupuncturists.

The years between 1870 and 1930, Burnett (1939, p. 23) termed the "Golden Age". Advancements in medical science made medical knowledge scientifically based and this increased public confidence. Pensabene (1980, p. 33) argues: "control of this knowledge gave doctors a degree of power and influence unequalled in the past". Researchers such as Pasteur (vaccination, microbial fermentation, pasteurization) and Lister (antiseptic surgery) influenced the new modern medicine. "Later in the nineteenth century, hospitals, laboratories and universities finally came together to produce modern scientific medicine" (Lewis 2014, pp. S6–S7). It is here that the seeds of medical dominance as we know it today were sown. These pivotal breakthroughs saw the beginning of the rise of the medical profession. In various dimensions, the medical profession has since continued to be successful in maintaining its elite position within the class structure and the professional hierarchy by control and regulation of access to healthcare delivery (Turner 1995).

## Medical Dominance

In his analysis of the professions, Johnson (1972, p. 45) concluded: "the profession is a peculiar type of occupational control rather than an expression of the inherent nature of a particular occupation". Professionalization for the medical profession has facilitated supply of quality medical care to the public, but it has also increased the control of the profession over the medical market. The rise of the medical profession in Australia has not been without struggle, however, and it has on occasions had to battle with the State. Professional bodies such as the AMA and before its inception the British Medical Association (BMA) have always resisted State intervention and guarded their control of fee-for-service medicine. The AMA also exerts control over its own members (medical practitioners). Into the twentieth century, the AMA/BMA fiercely defended the right to private practice. Keleher (2016, p. 397) suggests:

> So strong was the pressure on doctors from the BMA, that the doctors were reluctant to take on government salaried positions which were perceived as a challenge to the independence of the medical profession. Any increase in public provision was seen as a direct threat to private medicine.

The 1940s saw a battleground develop between the Chifley Labor Government and private medical interests. At this time in the UK, there was talk of the development of a national health system. Doctors in Australia viewed this initiative as indicative of socialised medicine and through the BMA strongly protested against salaried medical positions. Protests intensified when the Chifley Government proposed the establishment of clinics staffed by salaried medical practitioners. Despite the failure of negotiations, the Queensland government set up a free public hospital service. The State and the medical profession have a relationship often filled with tensions. The RACGP (Royal Australian College of General Practitioners 2010) advises that:

> In Australia today, medical practitioners have high levels of clinical autonomy in decision-making that affects patient care. That is, they are free to make decisions, within the parameters of evidence-based care, that affect the clinical care they provide rather than having these decisions imposed upon them.

Due to the fact that the health of the population is of major concern to the State and the professional autonomy and independence enjoyed by the medical profession, it is essential that the State enters into negotiation with the medical profession regarding policies and initiatives that are likely to affect the practice of medicine. There are, however, many stakeholders with vested interests in the healthcare system. Following Gray (2004), Krassnitzer and Willis (2016, p. 19) categorise these interests: "Service providers are concerned with profit, income and clinical autonomy. Citizens are concerned with affordable access to quality services and Governments are concerned with ideology, electoral popularity and budgets". There is much at stake here as health service provision is big business. In the years 2012–2013, health expenditure in Australia was in excess of $147 billion; $101 billion by governments; and $46 billion by non-government entities (Australian Institute of Health and Welfare 2014). There is also an institutional mix of decision-making and shifts in the balance of power occur. A level of structural balance is held by various groups across the system (Tuohy 1999). Health provision and reform is moulded by the balance of power between three groups. For example:

> Power might reside in the government with its authority, or the professions (particularly medicine) with their highly sophisticated skills, or the private sector with its wealth. As a consequence, the patient is variously portrayed in health policy as a citizen of the State with the right to free health care, or as a patient to whom a doctor provides the best possible care, or as a consumer purchasing a health product in a competitive market. (Willis et al. 2016, pp. 7–8)

Initiatives for health reform are often the site for tense relations between various institutions. The power differential of the medical profession shifts depending on the conditions of the proposed reform and always operates to maintain or further the interests of the profession. This may involve allowing some initiatives while negotiating to eliminate others. The introduction of Medicare in Australia in 1984 is a case in point. This was successfully introduced by the Hawke Labor Government, which at the time, did not have majority in the Senate or the Lower House. The Government was, however, able to persuade and then secure the support of the Australian Democrats to endorse the adoption of Medicare. In addition, the Labor party was in power in four Australian states and these states were keen for the Medicare legislation to grant them public hospital funding. As a result, strong political numbers meant that the Liberal Party, the market (private health insurance providers), the medical profession and patient groups were not strong enough to resist the Medicare initiative. In this instance, the Federal Labor Government had the structural power to enact the legislation. This did not mean that the medical profession had lost however and according to Willis et al., (2016, p. 8) the new arrangement suited the profession:

> the medical profession had become irritated by the way former Liberal Prime Minister Malcolm Fraser had incessantly changed the rules governing the previous public system, Medibank, particularly for those patients eligible for bulk-billing. Bulk-billing was seen as efficient by doctors because it guaranteed payment, so the AMA was not as opposed to Medicare as it had been to Medibank.

The adoption of Medicare afforded all Australians to access free medical care.[2] However, as pointed out by Duckett (2008), there are inequities in access to the system particularly in relation to socio-economic status. The Australian health sector, while at times subject to tense, political institutional negotiations, remains one of at least a degree of medical dominance, which equates to medical sovereignty. That is:

> Medicine is dominant in relations between the health sector and the wider society; doctors are institutionalised experts on all matters relating to health. State patronage for other health occupations has been historically contingent upon medical approval or at least acquiescence. Registration has traditionally been on terms acceptable to medicine or not at all. (Willis 1989, p. 3)

---

[2]Medicare is partly funded by the Medicare Levy which is paid by taxpayers and depends on income level. Low income earners are exempt. Public hospital treatment for Australians is free but a Medicare Levy surcharge also exists to encourage higher income earners to obtain private health insurance. This is a taxation penalty levelled at those higher income earners who do not have private health insurance.

The profession of medicine is not static, however, and change in, for example, the doctor/patient relationship has been noted by Dew et al. (2016, p. 8). In the late twentieth century, the medical encounter was hierarchical and paternalistic: "laden with power relations rooted in social class, gender and ethnic differences". Today, the relationship is less paternalistic and more participatory, where patients are expected to take more responsibility for their own health. A case study of the medical encounter (Dew et al. 2016, p. 11), however, also revealed that:

> The culture of clinical encounters can lead to interactional submission on the part of the patient, and thus to delegitimation of elements of patient concern that step outside a biomedical framework.

Some argue that there is more pluralism in health provision today. Coburn (2006), for example, believes that while medical dominance was pivotal to analysis in health sociology in the 1970s and 1980s, other actors such as the State, other health professions and drug companies are more visible and more powerful:

> The practical and dominant issues of the day have transformed. Major political battles today are over the form which a globally dominant capitalism is to take. These changes demand that we view medical power more in process terms rather than as an end state. (Coburn 2006, p. 441)

Baer (2008, p. 257) believes that medical dominance has been challenged over the past three decades by six social forces: the professionalization strategies of allied health professions; health has become a broader concept which emphasises prevention and community care; the State has put regulatory efforts in place to minimise costs and assess quality and effectiveness of delivery; Medicine has experienced a decline in authority as a result of media exposure of fraud and negligence; growing popularity and acceptance of alternative therapies and increased concern for patient rights. Broom (2006) mentions an additional force: the Internet-informed patient. In their study of a clinic setting, Long et al. (2006) found that emerging ways for hospital clinicians to work together were challenging professional hierarchies. However, they also assert that their results illustrate:

> The complexity and embeddedness of values of medical dominance in health workplace culture. While confirming that organisational and policy change on their own cannot shift deeply enculturated behaviours and norms. (Long et al. 2006, p. 507)

Perhaps in ways medical dominance has declined or is at least changing shape but I argue that in terms of the power to regulate and control IMGs, medical dominance can be expanded to include the unequal IMG/the system power relations. I concur with Broom (2006, p. 496):

> Notions of medical power and dominance have been deployed as part of broader critiques of doctors' control (or influence) over their workplace practices, patients, healthcare rationing, medical training and professional regulation.

In recent decades, the rise of managerialism has posed a challenge to medical dominance. Aspects of managerialism have infiltrated into regulation of medical practice (Germov 2014). Increased bureaucratization and subsequent managerial strategies place doctors in a more controlled workplace. For example, Sociologist, Ritzer (2008) used the term 'McDoctors' to describe 24 h fast food type clinics. Working in these establishments, doctors experience monitoring, evaluation of work performance and less autonomy. Australia has seen a move towards more corporate style control of health service delivery in general practice, particularly since the 1990s. This type of clinical governance while generally accepted by the profession has not as Germov (2014, p. 399) argues threatened autonomy:

> The influence of clinical governance was cushioned from severe medical resistance because the pursuit of accountability and evidence-based clinical practices were difficult to object to, and were ultimately promoted by some sections of the medical profession. …the existence of guidelines and protocols did not usurp or undermine the clinical autonomy of medical practitioners.

More recent attempts to reform health care have been developed in the interest of overcoming duplication and fragmentation such as the move towards interprofessional practice (IPP) which is aimed at improving interprofessional collaboration. It is hoped that through education and practice as a healthcare team instead of independent professionals will result in: "opportunities for a reduction in the number of tests ordered, time spent in patient assessment, and referrals" (Willis et al. 2016, p. 13). How much collaboration with others the medical profession is prepared to enact remains to be seen, as well as whether or not medicine positions itself to be the leader/dominant occupation in a collaborative context. The literature indicates that medicine would dominate.

Digital health technologies are working towards a more personalised style of medicine where eventually patients will have their treatment designed specifically for their needs. This will include devices that enable patients to measure their blood pressure or cholesterol. Medical practitioners can now access technology to enhance their practice and patient security. "E-health has seen widespread implementation of secure messaging between health professionals, diagnostic agencies and hospitals using electronic referral systems and electronic health records, which is critical for increasing the efficiency of general practice, and medicine more broadly" (Keleher 2016, p. 406). Future advances in technology, present seemingly unlimited potential. For example, Susskind and Susskind (2015) suggest the possibility of 3D printing various body organs, perhaps the technology to print cells directly onto burns, or imagine personalised medicine to the point of scanning a patient's DNA. The question is, will new innovations and reforms still see the medical profession as overall experts and the leaders of new ways to practise medicine, in other words, will medical dominance still exist and where would IMGs be situated?

Medical dominance over the professional regulation of IMGs is the central concern here. How this control is operationalised is of particular interest. It is possible to identify three modes of domination with respect to allied occupations, namely subordination, limitation and exclusion (Turner 1995). IMGs in Australia experience subordination, limitation and exclusion as do allied health practitioners. The medical profession views these practitioners as the 'other'. The system also seeks to divide IMGs into two groups of 'other'. For example,[3] the competent authority pathway clearly promotes one group of IMGs as more desirable and suitable for work in Australia than others. Dr W (2012, submission 68, p. 7) wrote to the 2012 Parliamentary Inquiry Committee linking inferior treatment to the competent authority pathway:

> For decades the medical system has maintained a two-tier culture where OTDs are treated inferiorly to their Australian trained counterparts … This dilemma has not been helped by AMC introducing the 'competent authority' pathway, psychologically perceived by majority of OTDs from the other countries that they are INCOMPETENT!

Autonomy for the medical profession is crucial in the maintenance of medical dominance. Autonomy ensures the profession an occupational monopoly that secures its dominant position in the division of labour. This in turn enables medicine to decide where others, such as allied health professionals, are positioned outside medicine, and the subordination of IMGs within medicine. The shape of medical dominance and the position of IMGs within will be interesting to track as we move into a changing future.

Susskind and Susskind (2015, p. 303) point out that not only are the professions changing but the future forecast indicates an incremental transformation: "… we foresee that, in the end, the traditional professions will be dismantled, leaving most (but not all) professionals to be replaced by less expert people and high-performing systems". All is not well within the Australian medical profession however. Alarmingly, the profession has a very dark side, a toxic professional culture. Perhaps medicine holds within, the seeds for its own destruction.


## The Toxic Underbelly of Medicine in Australia


Bullying treatment (such as the stark examples from the voices in chapter four) is not just reserved for IMGs. A bullying culture is endemic within the medical profession and can also be directed at colleagues at the same level, junior doctors and medical students who are Australian trained. Reports of sexism and sexual harassment also join the toxic mix. During 2015 especially, numerous adverse reports around medicine's endemic, unsavoury culture surfaced in the Australian media.

The ABC's 4 corners presented by Kerry O'Brien aired a confronting program on 25 May 2015, entitled At Their Mercy. Reporter Quentin McDermott reported: "A toxic culture of belittling, bullying and bastardisation is poisoning the lives of young trainee doctors in some of our major teaching hospitals" (2015). The program revealed first-hand accounts from young doctors trapped in an "entrenched cycle of abuse where teaching by humiliation is routine". Further, sexual harassment and sexism is also a part of the toxic culture. The story of Surgeon Caroline Tan is a case in point. Dr Tan refused the sexual advances of her supervisor and complained.

---

[3]This pathway is only for IMGs from: The USA, UK, Ireland, New Zealand and Canada.

As a result, her career in public hospitals has been impacted: "I find that doors are closed to me that would otherwise be open to other people, so I've suffered enormous detriment". Another female trainee surgeon told the Sydney Morning Herald: "Sexism in surgery humiliates me every day" (Medew et al. 2015). The ABC program also highlighted a chilling realisation from a young doctor which indicates that bullying behaviour becomes a part of medical students' socialisation: "In one moment I could just see how this all happens. Someone bullied him, he bullied someone else, and now it's my turn". Then Australian Medical Students' Association (AMSA) President James Lawler received a flood of reports concerning sexual harassment and bullying following the ABC program. He told Campus Review (2015) that he felt powerless and made an emotional plea to doctors to take a stand against these practices: "It can't be my job or the job of my junior peers at the bottom of the food chain to speak up because the hierarchy is too high and too strong".

In 2016, Ms B, then current President of AMSA, described to the 2016 Senate Committee one example of sexual harassment experienced by a female medical trainee:

> A student reported to me that they were sitting in surgical grand rounds, so that is when all the surgeons in the hospital come together and have an educational meeting. Someone presents some research to them. A trainee doctor stood up, gave an absolutely outstanding presentation—they had put a lot of work into it—and a quite established male surgeon was very loudly interrupting her as she went on, saying, 'My, my, my! Haven't they let you out of the kitchen a lot this month!' and various other statements about her being female … He laughed, and everyone laughed, and the head of surgery at a medical school in that city was sitting in the room and did nothing, as did everybody else. (2016, submission 10)

Sexism appears to be systemic especially within the surgical fields and within hospital contexts. Perhaps female medical trainees are discouraged from entering the surgical fields particularly in the light of the entrenched culture. As at 2015:

> Only 10% of surgeons in Australia are female. Less than 3% of female doctors are surgeons and less than 1% of all doctors are female surgeons. Among surgical specialities, women are most highly represented in paediatric surgery (29%) and least highly represented in orthopaedic surgery (3%). (Walton 2015, p. 168)

There is also a hierarchy within medicine, where surgeons occupy top spot and general practitioners the bottom. Further, within the field of surgery itself, some specialist practitioners such as neurosurgeons and heart surgeons are viewed as out-ranking general surgeons, who occupy the bottom rung of the surgical profession ladder. In her article entitled "Royal Australasian College of Surgeons revelations: Patients complicit in promoting surgeons' God complex", Harriet Alexander (2015), wonders if the Australian public has, unintentionally assigned surgeons a deity status:

> For every surgeon who has a God complex, there is a bevy of complicit patients. Nobody wants to know that the hero who saved their life in the operating theatre has a less than angelic personality. Yet the Royal Australasian College of Surgeons has discovered its ranks are riddled with bullies, creeps and bigots.

Following a string of complaints, The Royal Australasian College of Surgeons sought the advice of an expert panel. The draft report produced by the panel was scathing about the current state of affairs and delivered a stern warning to the profession about the future. The report found:

> Nearly 50% of College Fellows, trainees and international medical graduates report being subjected to discrimination, bullying or sexual harassment. It is inconceivable that anyone finds this acceptable or contests the seriousness and spread of these problems.
>
> The status quo will not serve the future. Individually and collectively, College Fellows must recognise and commit to closing the gap between how it has been, and how it must become. (Knowles 2015, p. 3)

High profile neurosurgeon and brain cancer specialist, Dr Charlie Teo has been particularly outspoken about the state of affairs in the surgical field. Dr Teo is the son of Chinese-Singaporean parents (his father an IMG) who migrated to Australia. Dr Teo has not shied away from sharing his own personal experiences and views via the media. These have often been honest and confronting such as the suicide of a colleague following years of bullying. Dr Teo has upset many of his colleagues and as a result, some have been quick to criticise him. Charlie Teo has been referred to as reckless and accused of giving false hopes to his patients. Dr Teo tells it like it is and many fellow surgeons do not like that. On 7 September 2016, Dr Teo appeared on the ABC program: "Anh's Brush with Fame" (Teo 2016) and while having his portrait painted, revealed a truth that takes the concept of professional solidarity to a shocking level. It seems that some surgeons will even deny a patient treatment to protect their professional standing and reputation. Dr. Teo is a pioneer in minimally invasive surgical techniques for brain cancer and takes on cases other surgeons deem inoperable. Charlie Teo, by his own admission, acknowledges that brain surgery is the world's hardest subspeciality in medicine, and in Australia, he is the best.

The following is his account of a colleague's visit to his office:

> I've had a doctor come to my office and tell me…and this is a surgeon I have a lot of respect for, he was asked by my colleagues to come and speak to me. He sat down and said: "Charlie you've got to stop doing this, you're really pissing a lot of people off." I said stop doing what? He said: "Stop operating on patients that others have called inoperable." And I go: hang on do you want me to say that a tumour is inoperable even though I think I can take it out? He said: "yeah." And I said OK, look at this X-ray, look at that tumour, do you think you can take that out. He said: "yeah of course I can." I go, well that patient has been told that's inoperable, so you want me now to call up that mother and say that that tumour is inoperable and I'm going to let your child die. And he goes: "yes I do that every day." Every day he lies so he doesn't piss off his colleagues and he doesn't give second opinions that are different to someone else's opinion. I've saved thousands of lives because I've operated on people who have been told their tumours are inoperable and they weren't.

It is difficult to accept that not only do bullying behaviours actually exist within the medical profession, but that they would go to this extent. It seems that some colleagues will in fact go to any lengths to protect their self-interest. It is useful here to take a closer look into the full experience of an IMG surgeon, Dr Richard Emery. This story also reveals entrenched unprofessional and insidious behaviours and the ramifications of those behaviours come to the surface in Dr Richard Emery's lived experience and subsequently, those around him. Relentless attacks by a few jealous, vindictive fellow surgeons on his professional practice led to Dr Emery becoming deeply depressed, contemplating suicide and ultimately leaving Australia. Dr Emery's (2015) case was the subject of a special report covered by the ABC's Lateline program. On the 3rd September 2015, hosted by Tony Jones, the program began with a disturbing question:

> Tonight, a story that raises some serious issues for the medical profession. Does the system of self-regulation overseeing surgeons in Australia work and is that system open to abuse?

Reporter Steve Cannane (2015) brought to life the disturbing chain of events in Dr Richard Emery's case. In the program's introduction Cannane stated:

> Tonight for the first time, Richard Emery and other doctors speak out about the culture inside the medical profession and how a group of senior surgeons in North Queensland was able to prevent him from making a living in Australia.

The following presents extracts from the program's transcript. Answering the call for the need of a spinal surgeon by the Townsville Hospital in North Queensland Australia, Dr Richard Emery arrived from France in 2003 to begin work. All was reasonably uneventful until, after five years, he announced that he was moving into private practice (Queensland Health medical officers have been able to participate in private practice since 1986). Dr Emery now posed a threat to the livelihoods of those surgeons already in private practice. At that time, he received a hostile phone call from Dr U, a local surgeon who was then president of the Neurosurgical Society of Australasia. Dr U (2015) informed spinal surgeon Dr Emery: "If you move to private practice, you won't be able to pay for surgery in no time. So go back to France". Cannane (2015) reported that Dr U had no recollection of any such conversation with Dr Emery. Nevertheless, Dr Emery went ahead with his move into private practice. As a result, three months later saw the beginning of numerous anonymous complaints. These led to audits of Dr Emery's work.

Dr John Stokes, the former Director of Medical Services at the Mater Hospital in Townsville confided to Cannane (2015) that: "One surgeon told me directly in private that I should run him out of town". Jealousy of Dr Emery's clinical skills and advanced expertise as well as the need to guard self-interest was at the heart of the fictitious complaints. A consultant in the rehabilitation centre, Roger Watson confirmed to Cannane (2015): "He was doing things twice as fast and procedures the others couldn't do and they got terribly jealous". Dr John Stokes outlined to Steve Cannane (2015) the scope of the complaints made against Dr Emery:

> There were complaints about his blood transfusion rate and we audited that and it was normal… There were complaints about his use of item numbers and we audited that and it was no more abnormal than other surgeons use. There were complaints about his complication rate, so we audited a year of his surgery.

The results of the audits showed nothing out of the ordinary. However, this did not mark the end of the campaign by his colleagues in their attempts to discredit Dr Emery and inevitably force him out of perceived competition. Cannane (2015) reported that a further complaint was made and the result saw Dr Emery reduced to conditional registration:

After Richard Emery had passed these audits, another surgeon made a complaint about him to AHPRA, the national body that regulates all health practitioners. That meant another audit and being placed on conditional registration.

According to Cannane (2015), Dr Emery then took the initiative to engage Dr Rob Kuru and Dr Bryan Ashman to conduct an independent review of 18 months' worth of his operations. Dr Kuru, also a spinal surgeon, explained to Cannane:

> The colleagues locally felt that he wasn't or that they weren't experienced enough to comment on the type of work he was doing.

Richard Emery arranged for the review to be undertaken by surgeons who did a similar kind of work. The review by Drs. Kuru and Ashman did not find an unusually high amount of complications with Dr Emery's work.

In fact, Dr Kuru (2015) told reporter Cannane:

> The data that Richard supplied to us when we reviewed the types of procedures that he was doing, they were appropriate for someone doing complex spinal reconstructive practice and the complication rate, we found, was in published and acceptable limits if you're doing that kind of work.

This positive outcome in Dr Emery's favour, however, did not serve the interests of the surgeons plotting against him. The surgeons used a presentation made to them in 2014 by Dr Emery as part of a standard peer review process, to initiate yet another complaint against him. Dr Emery presented the results of his operations carried out over the previous six months period. Yet, neither Dr John Stokes nor Dr Richard Emery, recall any major criticisms made by the surgeons who attended the presentation. Steve Cannane (2015) asked Dr Stokes about Dr Emery's presentation: "So Richard Emery's presentation did it have an unusually high complication rate attached to what he was saying"? Dr Stokes replied: "No. In my view, it didn't and that's supported by the view of the two AHPRA supervisors who had both seen the audit before". After Dr Emery's presentation to his colleagues, nine surgeons (including Dr U) signed a letter of complaint (one surgeon abstained). However, only five of the signatory surgeons were at Dr Emery's presentation. The Lateline program obtained a copy of the letter, and according to reporter Cannane (2015) it said, in part:

> We all feel that Dr Richard Emery's rate of major clinical complication was well above what would be acceptable surgical practice. As a craft group we have had ongoing concerns with regards to Dr Emery's practice, but the latest audit presentation is deemed unacceptable by us.

Not surprisingly, Steve Cannane (2015) noted that: "Dr U would not speak with Lateline on camera, nor would any of the other eight surgeons who signed this letter of complaint". Also noted, is the disgust and disappointment felt by Dr Emery in that four of his colleagues would criticise his work without even attending his presentation. Dr Stokes (2015) believes the sham audit process was deliberately used to target and discredit Dr Emery and commented to Steve Cannane:

He wasn't given a fair hearing. He wasn't given help, which you expect out of audit. In fact, the audit that was finally done was used against him in what's called - the term a sham audit, where audit is used to harm a person. The intention of medical audit is to improve care and this wasn't used in an attempt to improve care.

Unfortunately for Dr Emery, his surgical colleagues withdrew their support. This action meant that Dr Emery could not operate and therefore not practise. Dr Stokes (2015) told Cannane: "so it's an easy thing for doctors to do, to withdraw support and put a person in a regional centre at great risk". This situation placed Dr Stokes in an impossible position and despite the fact that he was appalled by the unethical treatment of Dr Emery, he was forced to: "tell Richard Emery that without the support of his peers, he could no longer operate at the Mater Hospital" (Stokes, 2015).

Steve Cannane (2015) revealed that Lateline also obtained an independent assessment of Dr Emery's credentialing. The assessment was written for the Mater Hospital by Dr John Quinn, a principal advisor to the Council of the Royal Australasian College of Surgeons. Instead of criticising the practice of Dr Emery, the report by Dr Quinn was highly critical of Dr Emery's colleagues. Communicated in the Lateline program via a male voiceover, Dr Quinn's (2015) report stated:

To undertake, assess and monitor spinal surgery at Mater Hospital Townsville requires cooperation, collegiality, peer support and professionalism from all those performing such surgery. Regrettably, these qualities seem to be lacking at your hospital at this time… This seems to be personality driven more so than scientifically or surgically driven.

As for Dr Richard Emery, by March 2014, he had become suicidal. After numerous complaints, sham audits, constant requirements to prove himself and his practice only to have restrictions placed on his practice, and now, without the support of colleagues, his livelihood and career were being taken away from him. Steve Cannane (2015) reported: "He headed to the top of Castle Hill, and in his words, was ready to jump". What came next in the program was the following poignant quote from Steve Cannane's (2015) interview with Celine Emery, Dr Richard Emery's wife. Unnerved by her husband's text message, Celine Emery knew something was wrong.

One day I came home and I got a text message saying, "Take care of the kids." And I thought he was gone for a run. And when I got the message, I understood straight away that he had gone somewhere. I knew he was running up Castle Hill from time to time and I really hoped that he was up there, I really did. Otherwise I'd - yeah. So I drove up there and couldn't see him, I drove up and up and I - and I thought it was a question of time. I kept calling him. He wouldn't answer. And I was really hoping it wasn't gonna be too late. And I found him. I found him and thank God, he was just sitting, sitting. And I told him, I said, It's all OK. We'll just go back home. Just go back home and everything will be fine.

Dr Emery and his Australian family returned to successful practice in France. Dr Emery has been able to get on with his life after his appalling treatment in Australia. However, there remains collateral damage fallout for colleagues who supported him (such as Dr John Stokes) and for his patients who missed out on his advanced surgical skill back in Australia. For example, Dr Emery's patient Michael Johnston, who, due to a rare condition, has a spine that cannot support him sufficiently. After previous operations that had failed, Richard Emery offered to repair the damage for free.

Johnson (2015) told Cannane that Dr Emery said: "I tell you what, I'm going to perform the surgery for you free of charge. This is my Christmas present to you. No expenses". Steve Cannane (2015) reported that unfortunately: "Michael Johnson was about to be operated on in March last year (2014) when Richard Emery's privileges were taken away".

Johnson (2015) shared his experience:

> It was devastating, beyond belief. I'd waited 17 years to get my life back. We were two months away from it happening and it was taken from me. We were basically the carnage. We were just left behind. And it's not necessary. And nobody seems to care. Richard's the only one that cares.

There have been repercussions for former colleague of Dr Emery's and medical services director, Dr John Stokes. Dr Stokes (2015) believes he has been targeted for reporting unfair process and has been virtually punished for speaking out in support of Dr Emery. He told Steve Cannane:

> In that same year, I was notified to AHPRA vexatiously on two occasions. There is almost certainly a link somewhere in that. I've had a good, long practice in medicine without any complaints about me. And I suspect there was some ulterior motive of stopping me being director of medical services.

Dr John Stokes was badly injured in a cycling accident that killed his friend. The accident was cited in a notification against him. Cannane (2015) stated: "So they even tried to allege that you were brain damaged, didn't they"? Dr Stokes (2015) replied:

> Yes. That was the most hurtful thing of all. A good friend of mine died, who I tried to resuscitate at the roadside. And I survived with major injury, but she died, unfortunately. And that was used against me to claim that I was mentally incompetent and should be deregistered.

Since the (2015) Lateline interview, John Stokes has been subjected to a further complaint, this time made to the Minister for Health. Steve Cannane (2015) raised the concerns of local Liberal National Member of Parliament, Warren Entsch who: "says he's appalled by what's happened in Richard Emery's case and wants the complaints process-overhauled". Warren Entsch was a member of the 2012 Parliamentary Inquiry Committee. Many of the submissions from the 2012 Parliamentary Inquiry and the 2016 Senate Committee Report form a part of the data set for this study. It is noted below that there has not yet been a government response to the 45 recommendations[4] of the report produced by the 2012 inquiry; "Lost in the Labyrinth". Warren Entsch (2015) expressed concerns in this regard in 2014. He explained to Steve Cannane:

> Unfortunately, I really got - I got no real response, you know, other than say that my concerns had been acknowledged. Now that was in 2014. Since that time, I've written again, I've sent

---

[4]The Recommendations from the "Lost in the Labyrinth" Report can be assessed at: http://www.aph.gov.au/Parliamentary_Business/Committees/House_of_Representatives_Com mittees?url=haa/overseasdoctors/report.htm.

that letter to the new minister, Susan Ley, and I've asked her to actually focus on this. First of all, we do need to get a response to those 45 recommendations,[5] and secondly, I was hoping that we could've kept Dr Emery in Australia.

Steve Cannane (2015) asked Dr John Stokes: "Is that fair, that you can have your fate in the hands of people who potentially are competitors"? To which Dr Stokes (2015) replied: "That's not natural justice".

Not only was Dr Emery's career adversely impacted, he was also forced to move back to France. The impact on his mental health, family, supporting colleagues and patients is immeasurable and ongoing. The toxic culture associated with hospital culture and particularly surgeons is apparently of grave concern for the Royal Australasian College of Surgeons. The college has accepted all recommendations made by the Knowles report (2015) and has embarked on a three-year campaign entitled: "Lets operate with respect". The role of the campaign is to raise awareness of an action plan entitled: "Building respect, improving patient safety" which has three areas of focus: "Culture Management and Leadership, Improving Surgical Education and Strengthening Complaints" (Royal Australasian College of Surgeons 2016). This current toxic culture is not a new development or a shocking surprise. The college acknowledges on its Web page that bullying is not confined to surgeons; it extends across the health sector:

> Bullying is a real problem for our profession, like it is in the rest of the health sector. Almost half of us have seen it or felt it. Now is the time to build respect and improve patient safety in surgery. We have to deal with discrimination, bullying and sexual harassment. (Royal Australasian College of Surgeons, 2016)

The 2016 Senate Community Affairs References Committee on Medical complaints process in Australia report raised vexatious complaints and the adequacy of AHPRA to adequately deal with them as a key issue. There was evidence that the complaints process had become a vehicle for vexatious complaints and therefore a tool of bullying and harassment. The committee report (2016, pp. 21–22) stated:

> The committee recognises that vexatious complaints are not always readily apparent, but is not convinced that AHPRA's processes are adequate for the purpose of identifying complaints made vexatiously. In particular submitters allege that notifications were lodged against them in response to their own complaints of bullying and harassment.

The pursuit of self-interest often underpins vexatious complaints. Dr K, Chair of the advocacy group Health Practitioners Australia Reform Association (HPARA), informed the Senate Committee that this is a significant problem for medical practitioners:

> These people [those making vexatious complaints] are misusing AHPRA for their own personal reasons. It is very rare, if ever, that AHPRA have taken action against people who

---

[5]I contacted the Department of the House of Representatives on 27th June 2016 re a government response to the 45 recommendations. The report was tabled on 19 March 2012. It is expected that governments respond within 6 months. The email reply stated: ..."You may feel free to contact the Health Minister or the Department of Health for a response noting also that a number of the recommendations are directed at the AMC(an independent national standards body).

have lodged vexatious claims. There is an absolute abuse of the mandatory notification process. It was put in there in the guise of being in the public interest, but really it is in the interests of the people making the complaint. (2016, p. 22)

The lengthy delay in dealing with complaints was also noted with the average age of open notification, currently at 137 days (2016, p. 24). Dr F made the following statement to the Senate Committee about his personal experience of the complaints process.

The AHPRA process has shifting goalposts for those under investigation. You answer one allegation and another one surfaces. Trying to defend one's position without knowing the evidence and its accuracy makes for a star chamber circus. (2016, p. 26)

Moreover, bullying within medicine is not unique to Australia, it is found in other countries too. Medical schools in the USA, for example, have been described as carrying out institutional abuse through soul crushing boot camps.[6] It is suggested that medical students graduate from US medical schools with post-traumatic stress disorder which has been caused by their training. The findings of a study investigating burnout among medical students in the USA showed that while students may develop resilience to traumatic events such as patient suffering and death: "students exposed to personal mistreatment and poor role modelling by their superiors did not demonstrate resilience but instead showed higher depression and stress" (Cook et al. 2014, p. 752). Further exploration of bullying behaviours within medical schools based in other countries is beyond the scope of this book, but I suspect that this could be endemic in the profession on a global scale. This is indicated by another US study on medical students which undertook a systemic review and meta-analysis on the prevalence of harassment and discrimination. The study highlights the extent of the problem: "Findings emphasise how common this problem is in medical training programs around the world" (Fnais et al. 2014, p. 821). The media has provided extensive coverage of the most recent developments regarding the toxic culture of medicine in Australia. While it is well known that some media thrives on sensationalism, it is difficult to take anything away from the stark reality of the voices who speak of lived experience.

## Medicine in the Media

The media and other impacted individuals via television, radio, newspapers, You Tube videos and other social network platforms have been quick to share the 2015 complaints and their views with the public. In her discussion of problem representations Bacchi (2009, p. 242) acknowledges the media as a significant political influence and force in how issues are viewed: "they play a significant role in governing co-constituting problem representations and influencing citizen subjectivities".

---

[6]The situation in the USA can be viewed in: "100% of medical students report abuse" https://www. youtube.com/watch?v=3G6zgGIPgc and "Why doctors kill themselves" https://www.youtube.co m/watch?v=qyVA+Z9VZ4Q.

Reporting by the media can be very powerful in its construction of current affairs. For example, the analysis of newspaper reporting of the Dr Haneef case carried out by Ewart and Posetti (2008, p. 13). The study concluded that in a climate of 'war on terror', border security and national security: "An over-emphasis on crime and security can overshadow significant human/civil rights issues and effectively bury the lead". The work of Lupton (1998b) and Lupton and McLean (1998) examines the role of the media in the portrayal of the medical profession specifically and subsequent professional image and status. The medical profession of course needs to be represented in positive terms to confirm the continuation of the profession's high-status position. In addition, patients need to maintain their trust and faith in the biomedical model and the professionals who practise it. Following discourse analysis of media headlines, Lupton and Mclean (1998, p. 956) found: "… doctors and the medical practice are the source of competing and diverse representations. While medicine may be portrayed as a fraught, conflictual and politicised profession in this forum, it is also represented as offering considerable benefits to patients". Comprehensive and frequent media attention of the Australian medical profession brings a personal and professional focus to media coverage. Germov (2014, p. 345) argues that …" the fact that they are subject to such great mass media interest also cements their position as an elite group enjoying cultural and social authority." Media stories with photographs presented the archetypal male medical practitioner and depending on the positive or negative content of the story and were portrayed as either demons in cases such as fraud and malpractice or angels in cases of healing and medical breakthroughs (Lupton and McLean 1998).

The most recent media attention, again regarding the RACS, demonstrates the particular plight of IMG surgeons who are from competent authority pathway countries. This pathway while appearing to favour IMGs from deemed more 'acceptable' countries does not necessarily mean a more streamlined pathway to recognition. In her article of the 22 September 2016, Julie Medew (2016) of the Sydney Morning Herald revealed another two concerning experiences, that of: London trained plastic surgeon, Dr P and American trained ear, nose and throat surgeon Dr Y. Medew (2016) suggests that the RACS is "controlling the borders to keep out highly trained surgeons from abroad". Dr P experienced bullying, harassment and discrimination while attempting to have his skills recognised, while Dr Y claims that a deliberate delay in his assessment proves making it nearly impossible for him to achieve fellowship within the mandatory 4-year period. Dr E, a colleague of Dr Ys, made comment on his experience: "At each turn there has been an act of retribution that comes with the process … It has been almost child-like in its transparency". The Knowles (2015) report commissioned by the RACS, called for increased transparency in the RACS' processes. This highlights an intriguing irony. Ultimately, it is the media's role to inform the general public, and in addition, it can also become a source of data for research. Workplace bullying, for example, is a key concern in the field of human resources. In their recent exploration of workplace bullying in the media, Ramsay, Branch and Ewart, (2016, p. 87) note the importance of a well-informed public with a view to enact positive social change:

Bullying is carried out by people (not entities), and it is only people who can devise policies and procedures and enact behavioural norms within contexts and processes that can
encourage or could reduce bullying.

Perhaps initiatives to reduce bullying within medicine on an individual level could
begin where the behaviour begins, by a move to involve engaging and listening to
medical students (Sklar 2017). When the voices of those who have suffered at the
hands of some misguided individuals within the profession, in the health system, or
in various associated bodies speak, it is a powerful voice. While medical students
are encouraged to report unprofessional behaviours in the workplace and are able to
access information on how to do so, such as the General Practice Registrars Australia
website (2017), they tend not to. This body also provides advice on how to be a
supportive bystander for someone else who is being bullied. It is difficult to marry
the 'social contract' proposed by Susskind and Susskind (2015) to the behaviours
exhibited by sectors of the medical profession. It seems that the profession does not
fulfil all the obligations associated with their suggested end of the bargain.

This chapter has explored the application of power and its origins in the medical
profession beginning with the rise of medicine itself in Australia from the 1870s.
Medical dominance exists firstly over medicine's work, secondly over the work
of other health practitioners and thirdly over society. Medical dominance is firmly
entrenched in the Australian health system where medical practitioners are institutionalised experts on all matters related to the health of the Australian public. It is
of a dynamic nature, however, and must adapt to constant challenges to retain its
position. The relationships medicine has with the State and economy as well as complementary and alternative practitioners has been noted. The medical profession has
the power to exclude various health occupations by denying them official legitimacy
and assigning them an 'alternate' status. This chapter has argued that the position of
IMGs within the medical profession and therefore within medical dominance is akin
to an 'alternate' status, an underclass.

A major concern is that the Australian medical profession, a profession with
considerable power, is imploding from within through a festering, toxic culture.
This culture, as shared by the voices here, seems to hold even more power than the
profession itself; that is, the power to destroy the careers and sometimes lives of its
members. Not only the careers of its members are impacted, however, sometimes this
toxic waste spills over into the public, the lived experience of patients. In this chapter,
the reader has been exposed to appalling examples of jealousy, self-interest and
deliberate, dishonest attempts to discredit colleagues. Bullying, sexual harassment
and other unsavoury behaviours have been aired particularly in relation to hospital
cultures and specifically the surgical specialities. How do IMGs negotiate their way
through this powerful yet less than desirable context? The following chapter attempts
to answer the fundamental question: What is the problem with IMGs represented to
be and what are the potential silences in the representations of difference?

# References

Alexander, H. (2015). Royal Australasian college of surgeons revelations: Patients complicit in promoting surgeons' god complex. *The Age*, 10 September 2015.

Australian Bureau of Statistics. (2008). *Australian social trends*. Viewed 10 November 2014, http://www.abs.gov.au/AUSSTATS/abs@.nsf/Lookup/4102.0Chapter5202008.

Australian Institute of Health and Welfare. (2006). *Australia's Health*. Viewed 20 September 2016, http:aihw.gov.au.

Australian Institute of Health and Welfare. (2014). *Health expenditure Australia 2012–2013*, 52; AIHW cat.no HWE 61. Canberra: AIHW.

Bacchi, C. (2009). *Analysing policy: What's the problem represented to be?*. Frenchs Forest, NSW: Pearson Australia.

Baer, H. (2008). The Australian dominative medical system: A reflection of social relations in the larger society. *The Australian Journal of Anthropology, 19*(3), 252–271.

Broom, A. (2006). Reflections on the centrality of power in medical sociology: An empirical test and theoretical elaboration. *Health Sociology Review, 15*(5), 496–505.

Brosnan, C. (2015). 'Quackery' in the academy? Professional knowledge, autonomy and the debate over complementary medical degrees. *British Sociological Association, 49*(6), 1047–1064.

Burnet, F. M. (1939). Changes of twenty-five years in the outlook in infectious diseases. *Medical Journal of Australia*, 23–28.

Campus Review. (2015). *Students want change of medical culture*. viewed 10 November 2015, https://www.campusreview.com.au/2015/06/students-want-change-of-medical-culture.

Cannane, S. (2015). *A special Late line report on a French doctor who left Australia after he was the subject of repeated anonymous complaints and medical audits—Was he deserving of scrutiny or was his treatment professional harassment?* Australian Broadcasting Commission, 3 September 2015, http://iview.abc.net.au/programs/lateline.

Carter, S. (2016). The pharmacist's unique contribution to Australia's health system. In E. Willis, L. Reynolds, & H. Keleher (Eds.), *Understanding the Australian health care system* (3rd ed., pp. 375–393). Chatswood: Elsevier.

Coburn, D. (2006). Medical dominance then and now: Critical reflections. *Health Sociology Review, 15*(5), 432–443.

Cook, A. F., Arora, V. M., & Rasinski, K. A. (2014). The prevalence of Medical student mistreatment and its association with burnout. *Academic Medicine: Journal of the Association of American Medical Colleges, 89*(5), 749–54, viewed 23 April 2017, http://journals.lww.com/academicmedicine/toc/2014/05000.

Dew, K., Scott, A., & Kirkman, A. (2016). *Social, political and cultural dimensions of health*. Switzerland: Springer.

Duckett, S. (2008). The Australian health care systems: reform, repair or replace? *Australian Health Review, 32*(2), 322–329.

Ewart, J., & Posetti, J. (2008). The reporting of the Mohamed Haneef Story. *State of the news print media in Australia*, pp. 6–13.

Fnais, N., Soobiah, C., & Chen, M. (2014). Harassment and discrimination in medical training: A systemic review and meta-analysis. *Academic Medicine: Journal of the Association of American Medical Colleges, 89*(5), 817–827, viewed 23 April 2017, http://www.ncbi.nlm.nih.gov/punmed/24667512.

Freidson, E. (1970a). *Professional dominance: The social structure of medical care*. New York: Atherton press.

Freidson, E. (1970b). *Profession of medicine: A study of the sociology of applied knowledge*. New York: Harper and Rowe.

General Practice Registrars Australia. (2017). *Workplace bullying*. Viewed 23 April 2017, https://gpra.org.au/workplace-bullying/.

Germov, J. (Ed.). (2014). *Second opinion* (5th ed.). South Melbourne, Australia: Oxford University Press.

Gray, G. (2004). *The politics of Medicare: Who gets what, when and how*. Sydney: University of NSW Press.

Johnson, T. J. (1972). *Professions and power, studies in sociology*. London: Macmillan press ltd.

Keleher, H. (2016). The medical profession in Australia. In E. Willis, L. Reynolds, & H. Keleher (Eds.), *Understanding the Australian health care system* (3rd ed., pp. 395–408). Chatswood, NSW: Elsevier.

Knowles, R. (2015). *Expert advisory group draft report on discrimination, bullying and sexual harassment*. Royal Australasian College of Surgeons: Melbourne. http://www.surgeons.org/media/22045686/eag-report–to-racs-draft-08-sept-2015.pdf.

Krassnitzer, L., & Willis, E. (2016). The public health sector and medicare. In E. Willis, L. Reynolds, & H. Keleher (Eds.), *Understanding the Australian health care system* (3rd ed., pp. 17–34). Australia, Chatswood: Elsevier.

Lewis, M. (2014). Medicine in Colonial Australia, 1788–1900. *Medical Journal of Australia Centenary—History of Australian Medicine, 201*(1), S5–S10, viewed 12 April 2017, http://www.mja.com.au, https://doi.org/10.5694/mja14.00153.

Long, D., Forsyth, R., Iedema, R., & Carroll, K. (2006). The [Im]possibilities of clinical democracy. *Health Sociology Review, 15*(5), 506–519, viewed 18 July 2012.

Lupton, D. (1998). Doctors in the news media: Lay and medical audiences' responses. *Journal of Sociology, 34*(1), 35–48.

Lupton, D., & McLean, J. (1998). Representing doctors: discourses and images in the Australian press. *Social Science and Medicine, 46*(8), 947–958.

McDermott, Q. (2015). *At their mercy*. 4 corners, Australian Broadcasting Commission, 25 May 2015, http://www.abc.net.au/4corners/at-their-mercy/6488010.

Medew, J. (2016). Australian surgeons accused of cartel behaviour to control fees. *Sydney Morning Herald*, 22 September 2016.

Medew, J., Hatch, P., & Lillebuen, S. (2015). Sexual harassment in hospitals a major issue: Doctors say. *Sydney Morning Herald*, 9 March 2015, Health.

Pensabene, T. S. (1980). *The rise of the medical practitioner in Victoria*, vol. Research monograph 2, Health research project. Canberra: The Australian national university.

Ramsay, S., Branch, S., & Ewart, J. (2016). The use of news media as a data source in HRM research: Exploring society's perceptions. In K. Townsend, R. Loudoun, & D. Lewin (Eds.), *Handbook of qualitative research methods on human resource management: Innovative techniques* (pp. 74–91). Cheltenham, UK: Edward Elgar Publishing.

Ritzer, G. (2008). *The McDonaldization of society 5*. California: Pine Forge Press.

Royal Australasian College of Surgeons. (2016). Viewed 7 November 2016, http://www.surgeons.org/.

Royal Australian College of General Practitioners. (2010). *Standards for general practices RACGP*. Viewed 24 September 2016, www.racgp.org.au/your-practice/standards4thedition.

Sklar, D. P. (2017). What can we learn from the letters of students and residents about improving the Medical curriculum. *Academic Medicine: Journal of the Association of American Medical Colleges, 92*(4), 421–423, viewed 23 April 2017, http://journals.lww.com/academicmed/pages/default.aspx.

Susskind, R., & Susskind, D. (2015). *The future of the professions: How technology will transform the work of human experts*. New York: Oxford University Press.

Teo, C. (2016). *Anh's brush with fame*, Australian Broadcasting Commission. 7 September 2016, http://www.abc.net.au/tv/programs/anhs-brush-with-fame.

The Senate Community Affairs References Committee. (2016). *Medical complaints process in Australia*, Canberra. https://www.ap.gov.au/Parliamentary_Business/Committees/Senate/Community_Affairs/MedicalComplaints45.

Tuohy, C. (1999). *Accidental logics: The dynamics of change in the health care arena in United States, Britain and Canada*. New York: Oxford University Press.

Turner, B. S. (1995). *Medical power and social knowledge* (2nd ed.). London: Sage Publications.

Twohig, J. (2016). The complementary and alternative health care system in Australia. In E. Willis, L. Reynolds, & H. Keleher (Eds.), *Understanding the Australian health care system* (pp. 207–224). Chatswood: Elsevier.

Walton, M. M. (2015). Sexual equality, discrimination and harassment in medicine: It's time to act. *Medical Journal of Australia, 203*(4), 167–169, viewed 24 April 2017, https://doi.org/10.5694/mja15.00379, https://www.mja.com.au/journal/2015/203/4/sexual-equality-discrimination-and-harassment-medicine-it-s-time-act.

Ward, S., & Outram, S. (2016). Medicine: In need of culture change. *International Medical Journal, 46*(1), 112–116, viewed 3 April, 2017, http://onlinelibrary.wiley.com/doi/10.1111/imj.12954.

Willis, E. (1989). *Medical dominance: The division of labour in Australian health care*, revised edn. North Sydney: Allen & Unwin.

Willis, E., Reynolds, L., & Keleher, H. (Eds.). (2016). *Understanding the Australian health care system* (3rd ed.). Chatswood, NSW: Elsevier.

# The Representation of IMGs as Problematic?

> The unfortunate person who émigré is the one who is blamed most of the time. Despite great cultural, religious, familial and national bonds he often has little choice but to leave. With this in mind he moves to the land of milk and honey where he has always the feeling of being a foreigner. (Malekpour et al. 2009, p. 281)

This chapter begins analysis, given the current context for IMGs in Australia. What is going on and how can it be explained? What is the problem with IMGs represented to be? Does the ongoing positioning of IMGs constitute a wicked problem, one that is highly resistant to a solution? IMGs as a community attract an enormous amount of attention, and they are the subject of intense scrutiny. In fact, a whole organisational network has grown and evolved around the perceived need to regulate and control IMGs. This chapter is underpinned by an investigation into problem representations and the teasing out of any associated silences. Initially, it is useful to briefly look at the positioning of IMGs globally and the associated ethical issues.

## IMGs Global Representation: An Ethical Problem?

The international migration of the workforce has become a part of the globalisation movement, which in itself has become the focus of much discussion and analysis. Migration across the world has been enabled by changes after the Second World War and increasingly since the emergence of the World Wide Web. Today, there is a climate of vast international exchange between nation states from ideas and technologies to goods and services and, subsequently, the international migration of the workforce (Toader and Sfetcu 2013). Australia, Canada and New Zealand both collaborate and compete in the skilled migration arena. According to Hawthorne (2014, p. 1):

> They have cultivated 'two-step migration', facilitating category-switching by temporary employed workers, and the retention of former international students. They have developed

© Springer Nature Singapore Pte Ltd. 2019
V. A. Pascoe, *Australia's Toxic Medical Culture*,
https://doi.org/10.1007/978-981-13-2426-0_6

substantial migration databases, including longitudinal surveys to allow constant monitoring and refinement of policy strategies. By 2014 Australian, Canadian and New Zealand strategies had converged to a remarkable degree, informed by the national and international research evidence. Each government aims to attract 'the best and brightest' in an increasingly competitive global environment.

In Australia, recruitment of past international medical students has become an attractive option, as they already have full registration. As a result, they avoid many of the hurdles faced by IMGs and are entitled to migrate. These graduates are often younger and more familiar with Australia's cultural norms.

The World Bank (2011) reported Australia as having 3.3 physicians per 1000 head of population. Australia has always to some degree been reliant on IMGs to fill medical workforce gaps. In rural and remote areas, IMGs comprise over 40% of the medical workforce (House of Representatives Standing Committee on Health and Ageing 2012). The USA, UK and Canada have also historically required IMGs to assist when there are shortages in the medical workforce. IMGs constitute approximately 25% of Canada's physicians (Walsh et al. 2011). In the USA, IMGs make up 23% of physicians (Hoekje 2007, p. 327). In the UK, 36.6% of physicians were overseas trained (Campbell et al. 2015). More recently, other countries such as South Africa, Thailand and Singapore have sought out IMGs. In some instances, IMGs are deliberately recruited or they are enticed via immigration programmes (Iredale 2009).

The supply of medical doctors varies significantly around the world. For example, in 2011, a wealthy country such as Monaco had 7.1 physicians per 1000 and a stable European country such as Austria had 4.8 physicians per 1000 (The World Bank 2011), whereas a country with economic difficulties such as Romania faced an acute deficit of physicians with coverage of only 1.9 physicians per 1000 (Toader and Sfetcu 2013, p. 126). The UK comes in at 2.8 practicing doctors per 1000. This number is below the European average (3.4) despite initiatives to recruit more IMGs to the UK. The UK falls below countries such as Italy, Spain, Germany and France. Laura Donnelly, Health Editor for the UK Telegraph (2014), noted that around 500 accident and emergency doctors trained in the UK have chosen to come to Australia to practise.

What's the problem? Many argue that there is an ethical problem here, with relatively wealthy developed countries enticing doctors and other health professionals away from less wealthy developing countries. This can have severe adverse repercussions, for example, in sub-Saharan Africa where the World Health Organisation (WHO) (2016a) noted that:

Shortages of physicians and nurses jeopardise health system advances in many low-middle income countries. Sub-Saharan Africa has only 2 doctors…per 10,000 people compared with around thirty doctors in high-income countries. Meanwhile rural to urban migration of health professionals continues to increase practitioner shortages in rural areas where the need is the greatest.

In addition, more developed countries lure doctors from other more developed countries. For example, the Royal College of Surgeons in Ireland names Australia as a popular destination for Irish trained physicians:

> Only one third of foreign doctors planned to remain in Ireland and the longer the time Irish trained doctors spend abroad, the less likely they are to return to Ireland. Australia is one of the most popular destination countries. (World Health Organisation 2016b)

In some countries, it is considered a good move for the highly educated, including medical doctors, to leave the country of their training to work elsewhere in the world. This is the case in Iran which, with 20% of highly educated individuals choosing to live abroad, has the highest rate of brain drain in the world.

> Despite improvement in gross domestic product there is unsatisfactory resource allocation for the most educated. The host country provides graduates with all their basic needs as well as offering a chance to fulfil some of the higher-level needs in Maslow's hierarchy.[1] As a consequence, migration is commonly seen as admirable by the elites of society, at least in Iran. (Malekpour et al. 2009, p. 281)

Source countries have invested heavily in the training of their medical practitioners with the impetus on increasing the numbers of physicians to serve the health needs of their population. The qualified medical practitioner is a valuable resource which is then highly sought after by other countries experiencing a health workforce shortage. Understandably, some countries appear to be more attractive places to live and work than others, after all medical practitioners are also human beings with likes, dislikes, preferences and career aspirations. This presents an ethical dilemma, that while developed host countries are effectively poaching medical practitioners often from countries with poorer health populations and of greater need, doctors should be free to migrate to any country of their choice anywhere in the world. Medical doctors also have human rights. The recruitment of former international medical students has also been questioned in terms of ethics, however, as Hawthorn (2013, p. 21) argues: "while the ethics of international student migration remain a matter for debate, parents rather than source countries have resourced their education". Some host countries undertake to not receive workers from underdeveloped source countries, but this is difficult to police. The World Health Organisation (2011) in order to provide a global response to health workforce migration concerns introduced the code of global practice on the international recruitment of health personnel. The code, while discouraging active recruitment of health practitioners from developing countries with critical shortages of health personnel, encourages collaboration between destination and source countries. Circulation migration is endorsed enabling the transfer of skills and knowledge to the benefit of both countries. This is underpinned by the principle of mutuality of benefits. The code (World Health Organisation 2011, p. 2) encourages Member States (of which Australia is one) to: "provide technical assistance and financial support to developing countries or countries with economies in transition that are experiencing a critical health workforce shortage". Perhaps mandatory compensation of some kind should be provided from the host country to the source country. A compensation initiative would be inherently difficult to operationalise and would require a distinctive styled approach.

---

[1] Maslow (1943) developed a hierarchy of needs pyramid model where he argued that human beings require basic needs such as food, water, shelter and safety before they can progress to higher levels of needs such as love and self-esteem and eventually self-actualisation.

In his possible compensation discussion, Smith (2008, p. 8) maintains: "It would require a high level of international cooperation between countries with inherent competition with fiscal and ethical agendas which would make harmonisation difficult to achieve". Nevertheless, the fundamental question remains as Iredale (2009, p. 42) notes:

> Discussions about compensation are not popular with receiving countries but the question remains of whether it is ethical to use the skilled human resources of struggling nations without somehow paying them back.

Some IMGs migrate for adventure and opportunity, some migrate for further training, while some flee unsafe locations as refugees.

## Why Do IMGs Migrate?

Most of the participants in this study were motivated by the need for relative safety and good education options for their children. To raise their children in an English-speaking country was important and viewed as enabling better life opportunities. Some IMGs had more lucrative positions elsewhere but decided to migrate to Australia because they considered their country of residence unsafe. Those IMGs who come from areas of conflict often have to leave everything behind and are unable to return to their country of origin. For example, Dr Munjed Al Muderis, a surgeon, fled Iraq due to an impossible situation. Dr Al Muderis writes in his book—Walking Free (Al Muderis and Weaver 2014)—that while at work in a Bagdad hospital, he was instructed by Military Police to remove the ears from three busloads of Army deserters. His supervisor was executed on the spot, in front of his surgical team, for refusing to do this. Dr Al Muderis, determined not to compromise his principles and as a result be executed himself, managed to escape and hid for hours in a female toilet within the hospital. Eventually, he found his way safely out of Iraq and eventually into the hands of Indonesian people smugglers who facilitated his arrival in Australia. Dr Al Muderis was subsequently detained in the now closed, Curtin Detention Centre. The situation was so dire; he did not have plans to come to Australia; indeed, he did not have any plans at all. To flee to safety and avoid execution was the only motivation.

Unless source countries can offer safety, stability, good education and lifestyle opportunities, the migration of medical doctors from developing countries to developed countries will be ongoing (Malekpour et al. 2009). The desire for safety in terms of a safe environment and the subsequent feeling of safety for themselves and their families was an important motivator to come to Australia for the majority of participants in this study. Life in Australia was perceived as a lifestyle free from circumstances and events which were considered unsafe. In contrast, however, interview participant Julian (2010, interview 1) commented: "If things don't go well here for any reason, we'll just go home". Julian was from a relatively safe European country and was not motivated to come to Australia by the need for safety at all, rather for the opportunity of adventure and to work abroad.

# Risk for the Sake of Possible Safety

Situations of political unrest and control, military coup, war and violence were mentioned by participating voices as constituting unsafe conditions in which to live and work. Consequently, these situations led IMGs to leave their country of origin. Colin (2010, interview 2) was motivated by continuing political unrest: "There were on-going political problems so we decided to come here". Similarly, Andrew (2011, interview 5) experienced political unrest but was also concerned about his country's isolation from Western societies; he commented: "Primarily because of the political issues in my country. We were isolated from the Western community. We wanted our son to have advantage also by education in English". Shaun (2012, interview 8) sought a feeling of freedom from the political situation in his country and had the advantage of knowing others already in Australia: "Mostly because of the political situation in my country and because I already knew people who came here. We wanted a better lifestyle, a brighter future … to feel free". Nancy's (2011, interview 3) concern for safety and fear of becoming trapped in an unstable country motivated her to come to Australia. Nancy stated: "There was a military coup in my country and continued unrest. We thought it was best to leave while we still could in case things got worse. I did not want us to be trapped unable to leave. The place was not safe" (2011, interview 3). Despite a higher-status lifestyle for medical doctors in South Africa, Tania (2011, interview 7) was more concerned about the welfare of her children and their safety from violence: "We came to Australia from South Africa where we were treated very well indeed, much better than Australia but South Africa is a very unsafe country where there is a lot of blood-shed and in my view not suitable for children". The decision to relocate yourself and your family to another country is not one taken lightly. There are many things to consider, and the decision itself may be perceived as an exercise in risk-taking.

If the current environment is unsafe and therefore perceived also as a risky environment in which to live and work, similarly the decision to leave for another environment must also involve risk. The participants in this study who voluntarily chose to relocate to Australia for safety reasons prioritised their personal safety and that of their families above other aspects of life in their country of origin. Bauman (2013, p. 4) argues however that: "Security and freedom are two equally precious and coveted values which could be better or worse balanced, but hardly ever fully reconciled and without friction". Medical doctors seeking safety in Australia is not a recent event; historically medical professionals have fled unsafe situations and come to Australia for a new life.

For example, a questionnaire administered by Kidd and Braun (1992) from the Department of Community Medicine at Monash University investigated the experiences of overseas trained medical doctors in Australia. One hundred and ninety-two doctors responded to their question: Reasons for migrating to Australia. Kidd and Braun (1992, p. 19) found that:

27 (15 percent) of those doctors had migrated because of political or religious difficulties or persecution in their country of origin, and 17 (9 percent) had migrated for the safety of themselves or their family.

They also noted that these doctors had not migrated under refugee status. However, 39 (19%) of the 201 IMGs who responded to the question asking under which scheme had they migrated to Australia stated that they had migrated as refugees (Kidd and Braun 1992, p. 11). Given that Australia is actively recruiting IMGs from around the globe due to a health professional workforce shortage, it was somewhat surprising then, when Colin (2010, interview 2) from this study revealed his inability to obtain an offer of interest from a prospective employer. Colin was determined he was coming to Australia, one way or another, and stated: "I sent over 100 CVs to places in Australia and not one response at all. So, I applied for Post-Graduate studies in Melbourne; a Master's in Public Health. I was working on this for 1 year and then they offered me a job, they said you can work here as a doctor, so I said fine". Both Rita (2011, interview 4) and Alex (2012, interview 10) were able to take advantage of the existing immigration agreement between New Zealand and Australia. However, they left an unsafe source country of origin to migrate to New Zealand in the first instance.

The majority of Australia's permanent immigrants without visas are New Zealanders who arrive under The Trans-Tasman Travel Arrangement. This arrangement, which is often influenced by existing economic conditions, allows for unrestricted movement by Australians and New Zealanders between the two countries (Castles et al. 1998, pp. 12–13). Schotel (2012, pp. 22–23) argues that all contemporary immigration policies are motivated by some or all of the following considerations: "National security, public health, national economy, social and cultural cohesion, balanced national demographics and rewarding favoured national and penalizing unfriendly states". Authorities often use more relaxed (e.g. waivers) or strict visa/admission requirements to reflect the quality of the relationship with a foreign country.

One would assume that in an ideal world a safe environment and subsequently the feeling of being safe would constitute a basic human right. What exactly are human rights and how are they enacted? For Bauman (2013, p. 76) human rights have to be collectively won:

> It is the nature of 'human rights' that although they are meant to be enjoyed *separately* (they mean, after all, the entitlement to have one's own difference recognised and so to remain different without fear of reprimand or punishment), they have to be fought for and won *collectively*, and only *collectively* may they be granted.

For those peoples around the world who are not empowered to take control of their situation and leave unsafe environments, Australia has undertaken to accept a quota of refugees.

# Refugees and Human Rights

Australia has an official humanitarian programme. In the interests of human rights, humanitarian refugees may be entitled to seek refuge in Australia; however, the number allowed each year is uncertain and depends upon the policy stance of the current Commonwealth Government. For example, in 2015, the Turnbull Coalition Government adopted the 2012 figure of 13,750 with an additional one off intake of 12,000 extra refugees from the current conflict in Syria and Iraq (Anderson 2016). A Parliamentary Services research paper (Phillips et al. 2010) states that: "Since 1945, when the first federal immigration portfolio was established to administer Australia's post-war migration program, over 8,000,000 refugees and displaced persons have settled in Australia". From 1788 until today, however, Australia does not generally have a good human rights record, for example: historically since 1788, the chronic neglect of the rights of Indigenous Australians and currently in 2016, the offshore detention of asylum seekers (including children).

The whole concept of exactly what are basic human rights and whether they are the same internationally is problematic. For example, as Schech and Haggis (2000, p. 156) point out:

> Universal application ignores the fact that rights are based on cultural traditions and may vary from society to society. Human rights tend to focus on the individual...this artificially separates individuals from their communities.... Moreover the focus on the individual fails to recognise the common oppression which large groups of individuals experience in many societies.

Moreover, Bauman (2013, p. 5), reminds that: "We cannot be human without both security and freedom; but we cannot have both at the same time and both in quantities which we find fully satisfactory". The Universal Declaration of Human Rights clearly advocates that human rights are universally fundamental for all peoples. For example, the first article of the declaration states that: "All human beings are born free and equal in dignity and rights …". Article 2 states that: "Everyone is entitled to all the rights and freedoms set forth in this declaration". Finally, Article 3 asserts that: "Everyone has the right to life, liberty and security of person" (United Nations 1948). For the participants in this study who fled unsafe environments, the ramifications of their experiences may have impacted on both mind and body before their arrival in Australia.

Post-migration difficulties can be assigned to three groups: "socioeconomic stressors, social and interpersonal stressors, and stressors related to the asylum process and immigration policies" (Li et al. 2016, p. 1). Feeling unsafe is liable to raise the stress levels of an individual, and IMGs are no exception.

## Safety and Psychological Stress

Perhaps arriving in Australia, already having experienced significant stress could be compounded by the necessity for vulnerable IMGs to place their careers at the mercy of the Australian health system. In their recent review of research into post-migration stress and psychological disorders, Li et al. (2016, p. 3) found that:

> Across studies refugees who are more highly educated and had higher economic status pre-displacement show poorer mental health outcomes after settlement. This may be due to the greater loss of socioeconomic status experienced upon resettlement which can contribute to settlement stress.

Iredale (2009, p. 33) argues that the questioning of IMGs' knowledge and skills from a source country by another host country has a historical background:

> Variously attributed to the non-transferability of qualifications and skills due to: different medical regimes; styles of patient care; types of drug usage and levels of technology; lack of knowledge about the quality of training in source countries; judgements about inferior training in source countries; absence of adequate language skills in the language of the destination country; and discrimination and xenophobia based on race and or gender. The outcome has sometimes been the unfair treatment of overseas trained medical practitioners by some countries in denying them access to the profession, confining their practice to certain disadvantaged areas and/or impeding their progress or career advancement once in the medical workforce.

It seems that IMGs are indeed perceived as problematic, and there are several parts to the representation of the problem. The confirmation that there are problems is firstly found in the various inquiries held over time which have been tasked to investigate and make recommendations in relation to aspects of IMG/the system relations and associated policies and processes. The inquiries have all arisen out of ongoing perceived problems and, the subsequent recommendations made, repeatedly mention terms such as accountability, transparency, efficiency and unfairness.

## Inquiries, Inquiries and Requests for More

Inquiries related to IMGs have been occurring for decades; some have not specifically focused on IMGs but are often the subject of organisations and processes that impact on IMGs and their professional practice. The Clarke Inquiry (Law Council of Australia 2008), for example, was set up specifically to examine the circumstances surrounding the charging and detention of Dr Haneef, an IMG suspected of links to terrorism. Inquiries usually conclude with recommendations and those involved are encouraged to consider and implement the recommendations. There is no structure or overarching body in place to enforce compliance. One notable exception to this, however, occurred in 2003 when the Australian Competition and Consumer Commission (ACCC) imposed twenty-one conditions on the RACS's accreditation processes (Iredale 2009). This was the result of a two-year investigation into unfair restriction to fellowship. It is beyond the scope of this book to delve deeply into every inquiry; however, the following are some of the more notable investigations.

The Fry Committee set up in 1982 is an extensive two-volume report that examines conditions around all overseas qualifications (including medicine). Particularly relevant recommendations in terms of medicine include that: "A formal appeal system constitute an integral part of every assessment procedure…and an examination of both portability of qualifications between States and the discriminatory nature of current reciprocity arrangements" (1982, pp. 7–8). At this time, assessment of qualifications was State-based.

Subsequent relevant inquiries include: The National Population Council (1988), the NSW Committee of Inquiry (1989) and the Human Rights and Equal Opportunity Commission's report (1991) entitled: The Experience of Overseas Medical Practitioners in Australia: An Analysis in the Light of the Racial Discrimination Act 1975. The Committee of Inquiry into Medical Education and the Medical Workforce (1988) (sometimes referred to as the Doherty report) was partially initiated by complaints from the AMA that there were too many IMGs coming to Australia. The climate at the time was one of concerns regarding: overservicing in metropolitan areas, the threat of competition and a Medicare explosion. The report resulted in a reduction of medical student places and a reduced intake into the RACGP (Iredale 2009). In 2004, the Australian Competition and Consumer Commission (ACCC) jointly with the Australian Health Workforce Officials Committee (AHWOC) (2005) reviewed the selection, training and accreditation arrangements of all specialist colleges. The 2005 report recommended: further consideration of the recognition of prior overseas training and greater transparency of assessment criteria. Also in 2005, the Productivity Commission and The Australian Health Workforce Advisory Committee (2005) tabled a report on the Australian health workforce to the Council of Australian Governments (COAG). The report's terms of reference included a concern with all major health professions, but it was noted that the accreditation and registration for medical doctors was overly complex. The Law Council of Australia's (2008) inquiry into the case of IMG, Dr Muhamed Haneef was associated with suspected terrorism. Arrested in 2007 and detained for 12 days before being charged, Dr Haneef was accused of providing a subscriber information module (SIM) card to a terrorist organisation in the UK and his 457 visa was revoked (see Clarke Inquiry,[2] 2008 (Ewart and Posetti 2008). There was extensive media coverage of the story at the time, and Dr Haneef, also a Muslim, was demonised. This linked IMGs to terrorism a connection easily made by the Australian public in conjunction with the anti-terrorism, national security rhetoric championed by the Howard Government at the time. Dr Haneef (now without a visa) returned home to India to await legal processes in preference to being accommodated in community-based immigration detention. The charge was eventually withdrawn due to a lack of evidence, and Dr Haneef's visa was reinstated by the full bench of the Australian Federal Court. The Commonwealth Government

---

[2]The Hon. Mr. Clarke QC, 16 May 2008, Clarke Inquiry into the Case of Dr Mohamed Haneef https://www.lawcouncil.asn.au/lawcouncil/images/LCA-PDF/a-z-docs/.

awarded Dr Haneef compensation of an undisclosed amount (Ewart 2012). In 2011, The Parliament of Australia Senate Finance and Public Administration References Committee investigated the administration of health practitioner registration by the Australian Health Practitioner Regulation Agency (AHPRA) (2011), a relatively new body at the time. It was noted that AHPRA's poor administration of registration processes had effected recruitment of overseas trained health practitioners. The results of what was referred to as 'teething' problems included: prolonged timeframes, provision of inaccurate advice and lost documentation. The Expert Advisory Group on discrimination, bullying and sexual harassment in their draft 2015 report to the Royal Australian College of Surgeons concluded that gender inequality was a central concern. The report recommended increased transparency, independent scrutiny and external accountability to be fully incorporated into the college's operation (Knowles 2015). The Parliamentary Inquiry (2012, p. x), the submissions to which form part of the data set for this study, begins its report: "Lost in the Labyrinth" by noting that a significant number of IMGs have become intimidated by the system and as a result were reluctant to speak out against the system. It was felt that IMGs, while generally having community support from those they serve, do not necessarily receive the same level of support from the institutions and agencies that accredit and register them (2012, Foreword).

The system was found lacking in efficiency and accountability with IMGs having little confidence in it. In addition, IMGs were faced with duplication and administration hurdles and subjected to discrimination and anti-competitive practices. It was noted that these have impacted the success of some IMGs in registration for practice in their chosen speciality. The committee recommended that red tape be reduced while ensuring maintenance of high standards (House of Representatives Standing Committee on Health and Ageing 2012). In 2013, The Victorian Government also held an inquiry into the performance of AHPRA (2014). The subsequent 2014 report by the Legal and Social Issues Legislation Committee of the Victorian Parliament investigated the authority for effectiveness, efficiency and fairness. The subsequent AHPRA (2014) media release states that "AHPRA engaged fully with the committee during the inquiry and welcomes its calls for increased: transparency, accountability and reporting to parliament". AHPRA (2014) also welcomed a stipulated forthcoming independent three-year review. However, seemingly resistant to change, AHPRA also stated: "We advised the Committee that we would be concerned about the risks of making any substantial changes to the way we work in Victoria..." Further subsequent requests for investigation have been made. In 2015, Neurosurgeon Dr Charlie Teo called for an inquiry into the bullying behaviours of surgeons (Sherden and Cannane) and also in 2015, then South Australian Senator, Nick Xenophon along with Victorian Senator John Madigan called for a Senate Inquiry into medical complaints. In a 2016 press release from Senator Xenophon's office, Senator Madigan stated: "Despite denials by AHPRA, I know of at least seven doctors in Australia who have been hounded from work through bullying and harassment by AHPRA". (Xenophon 2016). These inquiry requests resulted in the most recent inquiry that of the 2016 Senate Community Affairs References Committee entitled: "Medical Complaints Process in Australia". Senators Xenophon and Madigan were inquiry members. The subsequent recommendations of the inquiry were directed to all parties with the responsibility for addressing bullying in the medical profession: governments, hospitals, speciality colleges and universities.[3] The parties are requested to: "commit to ongoing and sustained action and resources to eliminate these behaviours" (Senate Committee 2016, p. x.). AHPRA and its processes attracted considerable attention from the committee from lengthy delays in dealing with complaints to inadequate guidelines. Professor S (2016, p. 13) commented to the Senate Committee (2016) on AHPRA's guidelines: "The guidelines from AHPRA are extremely loose. You could drive a truck through them". Similarly, as was the case for the 2012 Parliamentary Inquiry, many of the submissions made to the 2016 Senate Committee were either marked confidential and therefore unable to be accessed or marked name withheld. The Committee determined that submissions from individual medical practitioners or their family members which contained detailed personal accounts would be accepted in confidence. Most submissions were individual cases, and the risk of possible repercussions for speaking out was taken into consideration.

Another inquiry has been recommended by the 2016 Senate Committee to focus specifically on issues around the need to review the handling of medical complaints, patient safety and the National Law. I suspect that there will be further issues raised and requests for investigation made into the future. Whether or not these eventuate into actual inquiries or whether they resolve any of the issues raised remains to be seen. What is clear however, is that there are numerous 'problems' within and associated with Australia's medical culture and IMGs seem to be portrayed as 'problematic'. Analysis suggests that the current positioning of IMGs in Australia's medical culture and the system which has evolved to maintain that position has in itself become a wicked problem. That is why the situation will continue in its current vein despite all manner of inquiries into structures, practices, policies and procedures. What exactly is a wicked problem?

> A wicked problem is a complex policy problem highly resistant to resolution. They challenge our governance structures, our skills base and our organisational capacity. (Australian Public Service Commission 2007, p.iii)

The government is well aware of wicked problems and is constantly attempting to deal with them. Australian Public Service Commissioner Lynelle Briggs wrote in 2007 that many of the most difficult challenges in policy for the Australian Public Service (APS) involved tackling wicked problems. Wicked problems are characterised by:

> Social complexity, they cross the boundaries of APS agencies and cross jurisdictional boundaries. Stakeholders and experts often disagree about the exact nature and causes of the problems and not surprisingly they disagree about the best way to tackle them. (Australian Public Service Commission 2007, p. 35)

---

[3] The recommendations of the 2016 Senate Community Affairs References Committee Medical Complaints Process in Australia can be viewed at: http://www.aph.gov.au/Parliamentary_Busines s/Committees/Senate/CommunityAffairs/MedicalComplaints.

The innovative work of Carol Bacchi (2009) brings fresh perceptions to the wicked problem debate and advocates a post-structural approach to policy which asks: 'what's the problem represented to be'. Bacchi's critical rather than descriptive form of analysis argues that: "We need to study problematisations through analysing the problem representations they contain rather than problems" (2009, p. xiii). Wicked problems may not be the responsibility of any one organisation. Examples of wicked problems in Australia range from chronic policy failure in addressing Indigenous disadvantage to the challenges of climate change and land degradation to the alarming increase of obesity within the population. Wicked problems however are complex and according to Lavery, (2016, p. 1): "Every wicked problem is essentially unique and every wicked problem can be considered a symptom of another problem". These problems tend to be multi-causal and have multiple interdependencies and even conflicts within the wicked problem itself.

In terms of IMGs and the system, there are two key characteristics that are fundamental to the concept of a wicked problem in this context. Firstly, the power differential sits at the heart of the wicked problem. Professor Roberts (2000) in her discussion on wicked problems argues that the key consideration when tackling the problem is how power is dispersed among the stakeholders. Most of the literature supports a collaborative approach to the problem (Innes and Booher 2016; Newman and Head 2017; Waddock 2013); however, other approaches may be more effective, such as an authoritative strategy. The authoritative stance requires a particular group or individual to tackle the problem-solving process, while others agree to abide by the result of the deliberations. It is necessary then, for other stakeholders to also agree to the transfer of power to the individual or group appointed. The selection of the individual or group appointed may be based on organisational position in the hierarchy, knowledge and expertise, level of information or coercive power.

The second fundamental characteristic in the IMG/system context is the need for behavioural change. A key component of the resolution of many wicked problems involves the accomplishment of sustained behavioural change. It seems unlikely that significant change will occur in Australia's medical culture in the foreseeable future. It is clear that the process journey to accreditation and registration for IMGs is overly complex and the associated administration is cumbersome and repetitive. Despite ongoing adjustments to aspects of the system, subsequent inquiries and investigations consistently identify inefficiencies. The numerous bodies involved, their entrenched hierarchical structures and underlying ethos of maintaining high standards of health care in Australia make major behavioural change seem unlikely in the short term. Stakeholders may not be willing to relinquish or change their power status and may not be willing to change their approach. Moreover, a culture of bullying and sexual harassment, particularly within Australian hospitals in the surgical specialities, has led to the RACS report (Knowles 2015). One has to ask the question though: is an inquiry sufficient to instigate major behavioural change amongst surgeons? One would assume that these behaviours have been operating for a long period of time and as such become a part of the organisational culture of the specialities. Further, inquiries do not have significant power; they only highlight issues and problems and make recommendations for potential changes. Perhaps there is an authoritative, powerful overarching organisational layer missing in the system, or it is far more complex and perhaps too complex to fully address. Waddell (2016, p. 443) provides a discussion on wicked problems and advocates for a societal change system framework; he argues that: "There is a need for an agent with system legitimacy, power, and competency to nurture and when appropriate, push change initiatives to address…needs for a robust, coherent set of actions". However, in the context of Australia's medical culture which is already comprised of numerous agencies, the how of problem representation is more useful in the explanation of IMGs' positioning. Their representation has ramifications for how they are perceived and how they perceive themselves:

> How the 'problem' is represented or constituted, matters. This is because the way in which the 'problem' is represented carries all sorts of implications for how the issue is thought about and for how the people involved are treated, and are evoked to think about themselves. (Bacchi 2009, p. 1)

Bacchi's (2009) analysis framework of interrelated questions guides the analysis of the representation of the problems associated with the positioning of IMGs within Australia's medical culture. Bacchi's (2009, p. xi) suggestion for how to study problematisations is to:

> open them up for analysis by identifying the implied problem – what is seen as in need of fixing – from the plan of action that is proposed. This characterisation of the 'problem' is the place to start in order to understand how an issue is being understood.

Due to the nature of this study and what the voices revealed, it seems that much of what would constitute a wicked problem is indeed too broad, too entrenched, too stakeholder heavy and overall too complex to attract the ultimate goal of solving the problem. This is evidenced by the persistent problems found by the succession of various inquiries. The ultimate question then is: How can a wicked problem be tackled when there is a recalcitrant power base such as medicine, which is government-sanctioned, that sets the terms, processes and restrictions to further its own agenda? Bacchi's (2009) work: 'What's the Problem Represented to be approach (WPR)' is particularly relevant here. This is because the approach advocates a paradigm shift from a problem-solving focus to a problem-questioning approach. In the case of this book then, it seems that the terms of reference given by the government to the 2012 Parliamentary Inquiry is an enlightening place to begin. The terms of reference established by the then Minister for Health and Ageing, the Hon Nicola Roxon MP and referred to the House of Representatives Standing Committee on Health and Ageing reflect the concerns or problems as they were perceived at that time (see Chap. 2). The voices from IMGs and other interested parties were collected by the Inquiry Committee and constituted the state of affairs. At the outset, it is interesting to note that the Minister was very careful to acknowledge the two seemingly most important aspects of the overarching knowledge/power nexus: those of the role of the colleges and the need to maintain high standards.

The terms of reference given to the committee implied and set the tone for how the colleges, IMGs and the general public were viewed by the government. The terms constituted a deficit discourse which immediately established the Australian medical profession and the system as a ruling class, while IMGs and the general public were relegated to an underclass or 'other' status. The colleges were given the respectful acknowledgement they expect as the privileged custodians of things medical and the assurance and confirmation of their superiority. It was assumed that IMGs and the general public were perhaps unable to understand the processes involved and the decisions which were made; therefore, they needed a dumbed down or more simplified version they could understand. In addition, IMGs required assistance to meet registration requirements as they did not have full Australian qualifications which are superior to any other medical qualification obtained elsewhere. Finally, the standards set by the colleges must not be lowered to accommodate IMGs into the Australian system.

Discourse, in this case a deficit discourse which marginalises IMGs also informs our thinking. The medical dominance discourse which resonates from the terms of reference leaves no doubt about the power and control held over IMGs and the general public by the Australian medical profession. Kovach (2005) highlights the link made between discourse and marginalisation:

> the dominant society's usage of language to silence the voices of those who are marginally located... is the tool by which a meta-narrative of "truth" and "normalcy" is perpetually reproduced. In centres of knowledge production... the language becomes powerful and pervasive. (Kovach, 2005 p. 25)

The health system and medical dominance represents itself as normative, truthful and the custodians of medical knowledge. This is reproduced in the deficit discourse assigned to IMGs. The 2012 inquiry terms of reference are a clear example. In contrast to the 2012 inquiry terms of reference are the terms of reference given in the 2016 Senate Inquiry. On 2 February 2016, the Senate referred the medical complaints process in Australia to the Community Affairs References Committee for inquiry and report (see Chap. 2).

These terms of reference are not specifically directed at the investigation of issues concerning IMGs. As a result, there is not a dominant deficit discourse evident. While there is acknowledgement that the complaints process needs to be examined and that it must be checked against Australia's world-class standard of health care, there is an absence of a paternalistic tone and language. Also acknowledged is that Australia's medical profession does have a bullying and harassment culture by the need to investigate its prevalence. Submissions made to the Senate Inquiry (2016) from various bodies within the health system overwhelmingly claimed that their organisations take a zero tolerance stance on bullying and harassment (e.g. the AMA submission 9, p. 1).

The WPR approach (Bacchi 2009, p. 2) suggests that analysis take place with a focus on the following six questions. These questions, when considered systematically, guide an integrated analysis which highlights the ways political subjects can be conceptualised.

## What is the problem represented to be in policy?

IMGs have been problematised, firstly because their medical qualifications are not Australian and secondly because we need to maintain the high standards of medical practice expected in this country. This rhetoric runs through the policies and processes developed to address perceived deficiencies which could potentially undermine Australia's high standards of health care.

## What assumptions underlie this representation of the policy

It is assumed that IMGs possess inferior qualifications and poor English language skills. In addition, they are not familiar with how we practise medicine in Australia. However, some IMGs are somewhat more acceptable than others. IMGs from the English-speaking countries of: The USA and UK, Canada, New Zealand and Ireland are deemed more competent than IMGs from elsewhere; perhaps, the Australian public is more likely to trust a native English language speaker. These privileged IMGs are still not totally up to Australian standards however and must undertake further training and supervision in Australia.

## How has this representation of the problem come about?

As shown in Chap. 2, Australia has a long history of ethnocentrism, xenophobia and racism which persists today. As a result, 'others' are often perceived as foreign, suspicious or of less worth. The Australian way, our norms and values are assumed to be superior to others and amongst the best in the world; medicine is no exception. These social constructions are deeply entrenched in the fabric of Australian society and are not only reinforced and perpetuated in the socialisation of our citizens but also institutionalised, enshrined by laws governing our institutions.

## What is left unproblematic in the problem representation? Where are the silences? Can the problem be thought about differently?

The fundamental need for IMGs particularly in rural and remote areas of Australia appears to be on the one hand unproblematic. It is a fact that Australia currently does not have enough doctors. On the other hand, however, it is perceived as problematic that past government decisions have led to the shortage of Australian trained medical practitioners (such as cutting medical school places); this was negligent on the government's part. There is a dependence on IMGs in various specialities in rural locations. IMGs fill the gaps created by practitioners leaving rural areas. For example, in psychiatry as identified by Hawthorne (2013, p. 20):

> They compensate for an exodus of domestic psychiatrists from public sector and regional practice, who work in large cities in affluent suburbs, near private hospitals where they admit their patients. Rural psychiatrists, by contrast, typically lack access to urban amenities, quality schools and employment for their spouse. Many are on call 24 h per day, 7 days a week, providing mental health services in regions characterised by gross undersupply.

The silences lie in the toxic culture found within medicine itself, not only the treatment of IMGs but also the treatment of Australian medicine's own. Medicine's toxic culture, evidenced by bullying, sexual harassment, jealousy, self-interest and a preoccupation of market share, has been showcased by the media. It has been revealed via the voices shared here that in some instances medical professionals (especially surgeons) will go to any lengths to drive competition away. Dr Emery's experience in North Queensland is a case in point. These behaviours specifically were not aired as a concern in the inquiry terms of reference, therefore rendering them as unproblematic. Post the 2012 inquiry, however, medicine's toxic culture has emerged as no longer a silence but rather the elephant in the room. Moreover, recently the problem representations of Australia's medical culture have come out of the silence to the forefront of scrutiny. There is no real problem with IMGs as such. Rather, the problems lie with the injustices and inefficiencies in the system's dealings with IMGs.

### What effects are produced by this representation of the problem?

IMGs continue to be represented as a problem. This problem representation legit-imises the overzealous interrogation of IMG credentials. As a result, some IMGs suffer gross injustices at the hands of the system as evidenced by many of the voices embedded throughout this book. Some IMGs experience unskilled employment or unemployment. In addition, some IMGs experience adverse health issues due to bul-lying, exclusion and the inability to fulfil career aspirations. Also impacted by this problem representation is the self-esteem of IMGs and how they are viewed by the Australian public. Bacchi (2009, p. 189) argues:

> Members of outgroups-those located outside influence and recognition-are constructed as, in some way, lesser than the unspoken norm. Representation of the 'problem' sometimes produces a low sense of self-worth in victims of discrimination and contributes to the public impression of them as inferior.

### How/where has this representation of the problem been produced, disseminated and defended? How could it be questioned?

The representation of IMGs as the problem has been produced over a long period of time (as documented in Chap. 3). The problem representation has been extensively disseminated through the media. The drawn-out case of Dr Patel is a useful and interesting example in that, somewhat surprisingly, the medical profession eventually closed ranks and came to the rescue of an IMG. Perhaps, this defence was motivated mostly by maintaining the reputation of surgeons. The following extract from an article in the Courier Mail at the time read:

> Patel was charged with multiple patient deaths in 2006; found guilty in a 14-week Supreme Court trial in March 2010, before having the convictions sensationally quashed by the High Court in August 2012. With a bill for taxpayers topping $13 million - $9.7 million in special compensation paid to almost 300 victims plus $3.5 million in legal and other costs - Mr Moynihan QC said the complexity of the case, the defence's success with medical experts in court and cost outweighed the public interest in continuing. After eight years and $13 million, the state's top prosecutor has admitted the Crown failed to successfully prosecute Jayant Patel because it couldn't beat the medical experts the surgeon's defence arrayed against them. The decision to drop the charges sparked victim fury and set off a political storm. (Keim et al. 2013)

The Patel saga was active in the media for years. Panic ensued in relation to overseas medical qualifications and standards. Many of the processes in place today for the accreditation and registration of IMGs in Australia were influenced by the

Dr Patel scandal. At the time, there was a warning climate around careful scrutiny and increased vetting. Dr Patel, an IMG born in India, had arrived from practice in the USA and, because of this fact alone, was not thoroughly checked. It was discovered that Dr Patel lied in his CV and that he had been sighted for negligence in the USA. The defence has always been linked to maintaining Australia's high standard of health care. Medical dominance can be seen in a gatekeeping role to protect the Australian public from 'suspect' IMGs. However, silently and simultaneously, medical dominance is also protecting livelihoods from competitive IMGs, often via uncompetitive behaviours (Parliamentary Inquiry, 2012).

Certainly, the wicked problem concept continues to surface within policies and as a result processes. Why are wicked problems increasingly recognised? The Australian Public Service Commission (2007, pp. 6–7) advances some contributions while acknowledging that these only begin to scratch the surface. They include: the expansion of democracy and of market economies. Globalisation, travel and social exchanges may have highlighted value differences, weakened traditional authority and control mechanisms. In addition, technological and information revolutions enable more people to become active participants in problem-solving and as a result increase the complexity of the process. Information revolutions also increase the expectations of citizens for higher standards of living and therefore expectations that government should take responsibility for managing a greater range of complex problems.

IMGs do not constitute a problem, but are viewed as problematic in terms of their qualifications. In the interests of maintaining Australia's high standards, IMG qualifications are found to be, at best, comparable only to some degree to Australian medical qualifications. Why does the problematising of IMG qualifications exist? What is the origin for such assumption? The underpinning influences of problem representations are unpacked in the following chapter. This will unveil the Australian ideologies that conspire to relegate IMGs to an underclass within an elite profession. The positioning of IMGs globally and the associated ethical dilemmas have been discussed including the human right to feel safe. The reader has been able to gain an appreciation of from where and under what conditions some IMGs have come to Australia. The concept of wicked problems and particularly: What's the problem represented to be approach has been introduced as a useful framework for analysis in this context. Analysis continues in the following chapter where intersecting inequalities are explored.

# References

Al Muderis, M., & Weaver, P. (2014). *Walking free*. Crows Nest: Allen and Unwin.

Anderson, S. (2016). *Who will come to Australia*, viewed 19 October 2016, http://www.abc.net.au/news/2016-03-17/immigration-minister-peter-dutton/7254828.

Australian Health Practitioner Regulation Agency. (2014). *AHPRA responds to parliamentary committee report*, 1, AHPRA, Sydney, 12 March 2014, https://www.aphra.gov.au/News.

Australian Public Service Commission. (2007). *Tackling wicked problems: a public policy perspective* . Contemporary government challenges. Commonwealth of Australia.

Bacchi, C. (2009). *Analysing policy: What's the problem represented to be?*. Frenchs Forest, NSW: Pearson Australia.

Bauman, Z. (2013). In Z. Bauman (Ed.), *Community: Seeking safety in an insecure world*. Hoboken: Wiley, viewed 10 April 2017, (ProQuest Ebook Central) http://ebookcentral.proquest.com.ezpro xy.flinders.edu.au/lib/flinders/detail.action?docID=1187719.

Campbell, D., Siddique, H., Kirk, A., & Meikle, J. (2015). NHS hires up to 3000 foreign-trained doctors in a year to plug staff shortages. *The Guardian*, 29 January 2015.

Castles, S., Foster, W., Iredale, R., & Withers, G. (1998). *Immigration and Australia: Myths and realities*. St Leonards: Allen & Unwin in conjunction with the housing industry association Ltd.

Committee of Inquiry into Medical Education and Medical Workforce. (1988). *Australian medical education and workforce into the 21st century*, Canberra.

Donnelly, L. (2014). UK has fewer doctors than almost every EU country. *Telegraph* UK. 3 December 2014. https://www.telegraph.co.uk/.../UK-has-fewer-doctors-than-almost-every-EU-country. html.

Ewart, J. (2012). Framing an alleged terrorist: How four Australian news media organisations framed the Dr Mohamed Haneef case. *Journal of Media and Religion, 11*(2), 91–106.

Ewart, J., & Posetti, J. (2008) The reporting of the Mohamed Haneef Story. In *State of the news print media in Australia* (pp. 6–13).

Fry, R. (1982). Australian committee of inquiry into the recognition of overseas qualifications. *Recognition of overseas qualifications in Australia: Report of committee of inquiry* . Canberra: Australian Government Publishing Service.

Hawthorne, L. (2013). International medical migration: What is the future for Australia? *Medical Journal of Australia*, pp. 18–21, viewed 2 May 2018, https://doi.org/10.5694/mjao12.10088, https://www.mja.com.au/system/files/issues/001_03_230712/haw10088C_fm.pdf.

Hawthorne, L. (2014). *A comparison of skilled migration policy: Australia, Canada and New Zealand*, (pp. 1–14), viewed 1 May 2018, http://sites.nationalacademies.org/cs/groups/pgasite/d ocuments/webpage/pga_152512.pdf.

Hoekje, B. J. (2007). Medical discourse and ESP courses for IMGs. *English for Specific Purposes, 26*(3), 327–343.

House of Representatives Standing Committee on Health and Ageing. (2012). *Lost in the Labyrinth: Report on the Inquiry into Registration Processes and Support for Overseas Trained Doctors*. The Parliament of the Commonwealth of Australia, Canberra.

Human Rights and Equal Opportunity Commission. (1991). *The experiences of overseas medical practitioners in Australia: An analysis in the light of the racial discrimination act 1975*, Sydney.

Innes, J. E., & Booher, D. E. (2016) Collaborative relationality as a strategy for working with wicked problems. *Landscape and Urban Planning, 154*, 1–132, viewed 1 May 2017, https://doi.org/10. 1016/j.landurplan.2016.03.016, via Sciencedirect.com http://www.sciencedirect.com/science/jo urnal/01692046/154/sup/C.

Iredale, R. (2009). Luring overseas trained doctors to Australia: Issues of training, regulating and trading. *International Migration, 47*(4), 31–64.

Keim, T., Vogler, S., Tin, J., & Baskin, B. (2013). Dr Death gets off: Manslaughter charges dropped against Jayant Patel, LNP and Labor start blame game. *Courier Mail*, 16 November.

Kidd, M., & Braun, F. (1992). *Problems encountered by overseas-trained doctors migrating to Australia*. Canberra: Bureau of Immigration Research.

Knowles, R. (2015). *Expert advisory group draft report on discrimination, bullying and sexual harassment*. Melbourne: Royal Australasian College of Surgeons. www.surgeons.org/media/22 045685/eag-report-to-racs-draft-08-sept-201.pdf.

Kovach, M. (2005). Emerging from the margins: Indigenous methodologies. In L. Brown & S. Strega (Eds.), *Research as resistance: Critical, indigenous, and anti-oppressive approaches* (pp. 19–36). Toronto: Canadian Scholars' Press.

Lavery, J. V. (2016). Wicked problems, community engagement and the need for an implementation science for research ethics. *Journal of Medical ethics*, 10(10), 1–2, viewed 21 April 2017, https:// doi.org/10.1136/medethics-2016-103573, http://jme.bmj.com.

Law Council of Australia. (2008). *Clarke inquiry into the case of Dr Mohamed Haneef*, Canberra.

Li, S. S. Y., Liddell, B. J., & Nickerson, A. (2016). The relationship between post-migration stress and psychological disorders in refugees and asylum seekers. *Current Psychiatry Reports, 18*(82), 1–9, viewed 19 April 2017, http://cugmhp.org/wp-content/uploads/2017/03/The-Relationship-Between-Post-Migration-Stress-And-Psychological-Disorders-In-Refugees-And-Assylum-See kers.

Malekpour, M., Fatehizadeh, M., Hashemian, S., & Velayati, A. (2009). Retaining health manpower in developing countries. *The Lancet*, 374(9686), 291–292, viewed 2 November 2012, http://www.thelancet.com/.

Newman, J., & Head, B. (2017). The national context of wicked problems: Comparing policies on gun violence in the US, Canada, and Australia. *Journal of Comparative Policy Analysis: Research and Practice, 19*(1), 40–53.

Phillips, J., Klapdor, M., & Simon-Davies, J. (2010). *Migration to Australia since federation: A guide to the statistics* (pp. 1–29), viewed 23 May 2017, http://www.aph.gov.au/About_Parliame nt/Parliament_Departments/Parliamentary_Library/pubs/BN/1011/MigrationPopulation.

Roberts, N. (2000). *Coping with wicked problems*. Monterey, California: Naval Postgraduate School.

Schech, S., & Haggis, J. (2000). *Culture and development*. Oxford: Blackwell publishers.

Schotel, B. (2012). *On the right of exclusion: Law, ethics and immigration policy*. New York: Routledge.

Sherden, A., & Cannane, S. (2015). *Neurosurgeon Dr Charlie teo says 'bullying culture' in medicine destroying lives, backs call for inquiry* Lateline 4 September 2015. http://www.abc.net.au/late line.

Smith, S. D. (2008). The global workforce shortages and the migration of medical professions: The Australian response. *Australia and New Zealand Health Policy, 5*(7), viewed 6 June 2009, http://www.anzhealthpolicy.com/content/5/1/7.

The National Population Council. (1988). *Recognition of overseas qualifications and skills: Report by a working party*. Canberra: Department of Immigration, Local government and ethnic affairs.

The NSW Committee of Inquiry. (1989). *Recognition of overseas qualifications*. Sydney: Premier's office.

The Senate Community Affairs References Committee. (2016). *Medical complaints process in Australia* . Canberra. https://www.ap.gov.au/Parliamentary_Business/Committees/Senate/Com munity_Affairs/MedicalComplaints45.

The World Bank. (2011). *Physicians per 1000*, 17 May 2016, https://doi.org/https://data.worldban k.org/indicator/SH.MED.PHYS.ZS.

Toader, E., & Sfetcu, L. (2013). The medical migration: Experiences and perspectives of medical students for the professional career. *Revista de cercetare si interventie sociala, 40,* 124–136.

United Nations. (1948). *Universal declaration of human rights*, viewed 30 November 2012, http://www.un.org/en/documents/udhr/.

Walsh, A., Banner, S., Schabort, I., Armson, H., Bowmer, I., & Granata, B. (2011). *International medical graduates—Current issues, Canada*.

Waddell, S. (2016). Societal change systems: A framework to address wicked problems. *Journal of Applied Behavioural Science, 52*(4), 422–449, viewed 25 October 2016, (Downloaded from Flinders University) http://jab.sagepub.com.

Waddock, S. (2013). The Wicked problems of global sustainability need wicked (good) leaders and wicked (good) collaborative solutions. *Journal of Management for Global Sustainability, 1,* 91–111, viewed 1 May 2017, http://journals.ateneo.edu/ojs/jmgs/article/viewFile/JM2013.0110 6/1637.

World Health Organisation. (2011). *The WHO code of global practice on the international recruitment of health personnel*, WHO, viewed 20 October 2016, http://www.who.int/hrh/migraion/co de/practice/en/.

World Health Organisation. (2016a). Medical and nursing students' intentions to work abroad or in rural areas: A cross-sectional survey in Asia and Africa. *Bulletin of the WHO*, viewed 12 October 2016, http://www.who.int/bulletin.

World Health Organisation. (2016b). *Royal college of surgeons Ireland workforce alliance*, 30 June 2016. World Health Organisation (WHO), 12 October 2016, http://www.who.int/workforcealliance/brain-drain=gain/irish_doctor-emigration-chalenge/en/.

Xenophon, N. (2016). *Senate inquiry into medical complaints regime: Health complaints system under the microscope, Canberra*, 2 February 2016, http://www.nickxenophon.com.au/media/releases/show/senate-inquiry-into-medical-complaints-regime/.

# IMGs and Intersecting Inequalities:
# Class, Race and Nation

Attending to the perspectives and experiences of those who do not have power to make their voices heard is undeniably an important step for understanding social inequality. Indeed, these groups are often the objects of political debates, rather than participation subjects of democratic politics, and stereotypes about them are rife. (Choo and Ferree 2010, p. 137)

However and wherever this production started, it continues, in old and new forms, with old and new aims, using old and new infrastructural supports. It takes a lot of work to produce race, class and gender, which indicates a deliberateness to the enterprise. (Ken 2008, p. 158)

This chapter argues that the intersecting inequalities of class, race and nation help to explain why IMGs are positioned as an underclass within Australia's medical culture. Through the analytic tool of intersectionality, inequitable power relations are viewed as intersecting oppressions which conspire together to produce forms of discrimination. What is intersectionality? In the words of prominent intersectionality scholars, Hill Collins and Bilge (2016, p. 2), intersectionality is succinctly explained:

When it comes to social inequality, people's lives and the organization of power in a given society are better understood as being shaped not by a single axis of social division, be it race or gender or class, but by many axes that work together and influence each other. Intersectionality as an analytic tool gives people better access to the complexity of the world and of themselves.

Analysis unpacks intersecting inequalities and their roles, which weave their way through Australian society and its institutions to influence the positioning of IMGs. Through the analysis journey, it becomes clear that Australia's medical culture has been and continues to be influenced by deeply entrenched norms, assumptions, values and beliefs. The task here is to explore the social relations (structure and agency) between and within the fields/occupation of medicine in Australia particularly in relation to the IMG community and the Australian trained medical community. Following Hills Collins (2010), analysis is framed by presenting IMGs as an occupational community, as a community construct. The doctors share the same occupation/profession but IMGs are singled out as different, as the 'other'. Therefore, IMGs and Australian

© Springer Nature Singapore Pte Ltd. 2019
V. A. Pascoe, *Australia's Toxic Medical Culture*,
https://doi.org/10.1007/978-981-13-2426-0_7

trained medical graduates are also separate communities. While the profession is considered elite there are 'double standards' at work. IMGs constitute oppressed elite, in that they become an underclass while still remaining medical professionals. Analysis through class, race and nation explores the root causes which underlie the 'double standards' rationale and advance an explanation for why this exists. Many intersectionality scholars include gender in their studies. I have deliberately left gender, as a specific intersecting inequality, out of this analysis. I acknowledge the importance of gender analysis, but in this case, I did not want to divide the IMG community on a gender basis nor in any way further disempower the IMG community, preferring to keep their solidarity as purely a professional community. As Sefa Dei (2008, p. 81) notes:

> It is indeed crucial and strategic that in intersectional discursive politics we look for a common lens of identity construction which allows multiple parties to join in a community of shared purpose.

Further, a thorough analysis of gender as an intersecting inequality is beyond the scope of this book. It is class, race and nation that most effectively aid in the 'why' analysis of the position of IMGs. Initially, the analysis tool of intersectionality will be defined followed by an exploration of the complex expressions of inequality. The role of this chapter then is to investigate more recent and ongoing examples of what has become the Australian nation: the prejudices, the exclusions, the violations of human rights, in other words, the more ugly side of the land of milk and honey. For these, reveal the environment for the socialisation of Australia's citizens and the impetus of Australia's governments, laws and institutions.

## Intersectionality as an Analytic Tool

Intersectionality was conceived by feminist, Kimberlé Crenshaw, a critical race scholar (1989) and followed by Hill Collins (1990). These feminists were particularly interested in the multiple oppressions experienced by women of colour in the United States. Since then, intersectionality has become central to many feminist works. It is essentially a tool for the analysis of the ways hierarchies are constructed and intersect allowing some groups to have privilege over other groups. The categories advanced here class, race and nation do not have rigid boundaries, however, and the struggles and injustices within are not confined; intersectionality is a flexible theoretical framework. According to Lutz et al. (2011, p. 132): "different forms of social inequality, oppression and discrimination interact and overlap in multidimensional ways. That is, the categories are co-constitutive and synergistic; no category has a single, fixed meaning". This structure can be viewed as "web-like" (Fraser and Taylor 2016).

The foundations of analysis have been set down in preceding chapters where the investigation of power practices via the study of processes and systems and the creation of systemic power have been explored. How this power is created, recreated and maintained in this study is via relations between the health system (the controlling medical bureaucracy) and the 'other' (IMGs: oppressed elite). Interlocking systems of oppression are part of a single, historically created system. Against a background of institutional power, a deliberate exclusion via tactics of roadblocks, lengthy delays and other strategies for control, make the process to full medical registration for IMGs as difficult as possible. This study is also a political critique of the social world which includes the relationship between power and knowledge and the experiences of marginalised voices, those shared with the reader from the lived experience of IMGs. The work of an intersectionality approach endeavours to confront power. The fundamental focus which underpins this book seeks to move to empowerment linked to analysis of power relations and the ongoing acknowledgement of systemic oppressions. Following Brown and Strega (2005, p. 10):

> By centering questions of whose interests are served not only by research products but also in research processes, it challenges existing relations of dominance and subordination and offers a basis for political action.

Unjust power relations and how they are created and maintained have been the focus for many scholars. Historically, classical theorists such as Marx and Weber, followed by Foucault, have been interested in the analysis of the relationship between the social system (structures, institutions, historical processes) and the social actor (discourses, actions, and meanings) and the organisation of knowledge and power. Foucauldian archaeology (1972), for example, seeks to unearth assumed thought. Bacchi (2009, p. 5) argues that: "this kind of analysis includes a search for deep-seated cultural values—a kind of social unconscious—that underpins a problem representation". Power relations in Australia underpin the focus in this case.

From a Peace Studies perspective, the concept of violence in power relations is useful in the case of the IMG experience in Australia; in particular their interaction with aspects of the system, which in itself is a manifestation of Australian 'normalcy'. The work of Savitch (1975) in terms of systemic bias and the work of Galtung (1970) in terms of structural violence, as well as his concept of cultural violence (1990) provides a helpful way to view how IMGs are situated and how power relations and the associated discourses are structurally entrenched in Australian society.

Structural violence can be seen as violence built into the social order. In his development of this concept, Galtung (1990) expanded his ideas to cultural violence. This perception of violence consists of " any aspect of a culture that can be used to legitimize violence in its direct or structured form" (p. 291). For example, distinct from direct violence and the violence built into the structure of society, symbolic violence built into a society's culture does not wound or kill but can be used to legitimize either or both. In addition, Eckermann et al. (2006, p. 64) introduced the idea of systemic frustration of aspirations which maintains that:

> the predominant social order denies one category of persons access to the prerequisites of effective participation in a system developed and controlled by powerful interest groups…- further, it is argued, the controlling groups generally define legitimate pathways to effective participation in order to maintain their own power.

In the quest to confront power and the agents who enact it, it is also necessary to consider IMG agency within intersecting oppressions. Black feminist thought offers an invaluable contribution to intersectionality and research concerning the marginalised. The work of Patricia Hill Collins, for example, advocates the significance of knowledge in a politics of empowerment and argues that Black feminist thought requires a paradigm shift in the analysis of unjust power relations: "By embracing a paradigm of intersecting oppressions of race, class, gender, sexuality and nation, as well as Black women's individual and collective agency within them" (Hill Collins 2000, p. 273). While intersectionality is strongly connected with women and gender studies it is not confined there, rather it has become multi-disciplinary and usefully utilised in varied studies that seek to explore power relations. Intersectionality has become a strong vehicle for critical inquiry and praxis (Hill Collins and Bilge 2016).

To assist in the investigation of power in this study, it is necessary to explore the influences which underpin Australian society that in turn contribute to the formation of ideas and their execution through the fabric of individuals, institutions and governments. This analysis is essentially a search for the 'why' of IMG positioning as the 'how' has already been revealed in terms of medical dominance (see Willis 1989). However, Bacchi (2009, p. 5) suggests: "The question becomes not why something happens but how is it possible for something to happen". This is a valid point and I note that perhaps the whole 'how' has not been considered. Perhaps the 'why' analysis offered here will actually complete the 'how'.


## Class, Race and Nation as Intersecting Oppressions

Intersectionality is a flexible framework and intersecting oppressions overlap. Therefore, the discussion offered here will reflect the connectedness of the intersections. Initially though it is important to note the interpretation dilemmas of the term inequality and the somewhat problematic oppressed and oppressor binary. The term equality has taken on the general meaning of treating all people in the same way and the term equal opportunity is now the dominant equality discourse in Western industrialised countries. This implies that individuals should have the same chance to pursue opportunities and have equal access to opportunities. This sits on specific meanings of inequality. However, Bacchi (2009, p. 180) argues that: "No term is more contested than inequality. It plays a key role in Western public policy, policy affected by Western laws and Western precedents by a set of binaries: equality/difference, sameness/difference, equal treatment/different treatment, equal opportunity/equal results or outcomes". Australia prides itself on being a country where equal opportunity is almost a given. In reality, however, this is not the case, racial inequality, for example, is clearly evident in Indigenous Australian communities.

In addition, the discourse of intersections can pose intellectual dangers in terms of the oppressor and oppressed status. In his discussion of race, difference and the discourse of intersectionality, Sefa Dei (2008, p. 85) notes:

Sources of identity complicate our understanding of oppressions beyond the oppressed/oppressor binary. Context, location and historical specificities themselves add complexity not only to our analysis of the intersectional and/or interlocking nature of oppressions, but also to essentialist claims.

Australia as context and location has indeed specific historical archaeology that is not only complex but often incongruent with the Australian image portrayed to the rest of the world. Australia is an imagined society and nation, and there are generalised 'truths' as well as contestation and conflict over what constitutes the Australian nation (Plage et al. 2016). Is Australia a fair and just egalitarian society or is it exclusionary and racist? Is Australia multicultural, or British/Western, or a second America? Is it an old or a young country? Essentially, as White (1997, p. 13) suggests:

'Australia' exists pre-eminently as an idea. While it has a real existence as a geographical space with defined boundaries, and as a political entity, a nation-state organised for the pursuit of political power. 'Australia' for the most part is something we carry around in our heads.

The political climate in Australia is a useful place to begin discussion around the intersections of class, race and nation and the positioning of IMGs. Governments pass legislation of ideas and processes into laws, and subsequently into institutional structures. The voters of the nation, Australia's citizens, elect the government. The government and the Australian voters should provide an image of what Australia stands for or hopes to stand for. A particularly interesting politician of recent times is Pauline Hanson and her right wing, conservative platform One Nation Party. Hanson declares that 'political correctness' threatens Australia's identity. The policies developed by this party and the fact that people vote for them demonstrates that a significant number of Australians hold racist and xenophobic views as well as an ethnocentric view of what constitutes the nation Australia.

## The Rise and Fall and Resurrection of Hanson: 'I Am Fed Up'!

On 10 November 2016, Pauline Hanson shared a bottle of champagne on the front lawns of parliament house in Canberra with her colleagues in celebration of Donald Trump's election to the presidency of the USA, which he intends to: 'make great again.' Hanson (2016) explained:

Why I'm celebrating is that I can see that people … around the world are saying, 'We've had enough of the establishment,' she said. Give people the power back to have their own democracy. I think Donald Trump will bring that to America and I can see in Donald Trump a lot of me and what I stand for in Australia. I think it's great. (Le Messurier 2016)

In 1996 Pauline Hanson, fish and chip shop owner, came out of political obscurity into the public spotlight and was unexpectedly elected to the House of Representatives as an independent. Her beliefs and ideas shocked 'fair' minded Australians and unearthed some others who secretly agreed with her xenophobic and racist statements giving them a chance to 'come out'. The media capitalised on her ignorance and ill-informed opinions. Initially, it was Asians which Hanson demonised the most, claiming that Australia would be swamped by them. Indigenous Australians also came under fire. Referring to Indigenous Australians in her maiden speech to Federal Parliament in September 1996, she ignorantly stated:

> I am fed up with being told, 'This is our land'. Well, where the hell do I go? I was born here, and so were my parents and children. I will work beside anyone and they will be my equal but I draw the line when told I must pay and continue paying for something that happened over 200 years ago. Like most Australians, I worked for my land; no-one gave it to me. (Museum Victoria 1996)

Hanson also mentioned that she was tired of Aboriginal people being presented as the most disadvantaged group in Australia. In the 1998 federal election, Hanson lost her seat but assured Australia that she would be back. She contested several state and federal elections as an Independent and then rejoined One Nation in 2013 and again became leader. Throughout her political career, Hanson has singled out many groups of people for undeserving criticism, such as claims that Africans come to Australia spreading disease, she was referring to HIV Aids (Museum Victoria 1996). Currently, Pauline Hanson is more focussed on the demonisation of Muslims. In 2016 after a successful campaign entitled: 'Fed Up', Hanson was back, this time elected as a Queensland senator. In her maiden speech, during which senators from the Greens party walked out in protest, she predicted:

> Have no doubt that we will be living under sharia law and treated as second-class citizens with second-class rights if we keep heading down the path with the attitude, 'She'll be right, mate'…Therefore, I call for stopping further Muslim immigration and banning the burqa…(Sydney Morning Herald 2016).

The policies of the One Nation Party (2016) include the desire to abolish multi-culturalism and the Racial Discrimination Act, promote assimilation, nationalism, loyalty and pride in being Australian. The party also wishes to withdraw from United Nations treaties on migration and refugees that conflict with our sovereign rights and laws (One Nation Party 2016).

It has been a long journey for Hanson, in 2003, a Brisbane court found her guilty of electoral fraud which was subsequently overturned by a Queensland court of appeal. However, she spent the eleven weeks prior to the appeal being heard, in prison. From her first appearance in Canberra in 1997 until today she has continued her populist public commentary and received a growing level of support. Pauline Hanson is not alone.

## 'Love Trumps Hate' and 'The European Union Has Failed Us All'

The election of Donald Trump in the USA in 2016 is indicative of an ailing economy, high unemployment and an angry working-class backlash. Like Pauline Hanson, Donald Trump's proposed policies range from ambitious and naïve, to exclusionary and racist, to outrageous and include: The proposed construction of a wall along the Mexican border and to detain and then deport all illegal immigrants. As long as the threat of Islamic State persists, Trump vows to stop muslim immigration into the USA and he also intends to increase defence spending. As a seemingly true champion of the working class, Trump aims to create a dynamic booming economy that will create 25 million jobs over the next decade especially in construction and steel manufacturing via an ambitious increase in spending on infrastructure. Trump promises to cut individual and corporate taxes while endeavouring to reduce or eliminate most deductions and loopholes available to the very rich (Poliplatform 2016). These policy initiatives may seem like salvation for a weary section of the American public, however, some policies may cause adverse reactions from other countries.

As Phillips (2016) warns in his *Guardian* article about the possible tit-for-tat ramifications of Trump's proposed 45% tariff on Chinese imports:

> A batch of Boeing orders will be replaced by Airbus. US auto and iPhone sales in China will suffer a setback, and US soybean and maize imports will be halted. China can also limit the number of Chinese students studying in the US.

Many Americans were shocked with the election result, and there have been protests across the country with the 'not my president' placard a dominant image. In an opinion piece, Ernst (2016) identified Trump supporters and a desire to go back to past 'better' times: "what differentiates Trump's supporters is their resentment towards immigrants, African Americans and feminists—anyone who challenges the hierarchies that reigned back when America was great". Similarly, the political right has been at work in the UK with the successful vote for Britain to leave the European Union (Brexit) in 2016.

The desire to return to a past which is perceived as somehow a time when a nation was 'great' resonates in this context. In a news article entitled who is UKIP leader Nigel Farage?, Chang (2016) writes of a nostalgic great nation sentiment:

> His straight-talking, man-on-the-street style resonates with many older, white, blue collar voters and is reminiscent of a bygone era when the economy felt stronger, immigration was lower and Britain was great.

Nigel Farage, a former Conservative, left the party in 1992 when Britain signed the Maastricht Treaty. The treaty led to the formation of the European Union (EU) and the creation of the Euro currency. Although Farage was not part of the official 'leave campaign', he was an enthusiastic and tireless campaigner and his party: UK Independence Party (UKIP) which he founded in 1993 had a mandate to move Britain away from Europe. During the leave campaign, Farage toured nationwide in the 'battle bus'. The UKIP has become a force in British politics even though the party only has one Member of Parliament in the House of Commons and despite former Prime Minister David Cameron's opinion of the party as: "fruitcakes, loonies and closet racists"(Chang 2016). Farage has never been able to secure a seat in the UK parliament but in 1999 successfully gained a seat in the European parliament. The impetus to leave the EU was also closely linked to immigration and Farage made no secret of his xenophobic views. The UKIP poster entitled: "Breaking Point The EU Has Failed Us All" featured the image of a long queue of migrants entering Europe in 2015. This initiative attracted many critics, and he was accused of promoting racist and xenophobic views (Armstrong and Britton 2016). Farage has publicly backed Australia's tough immigration policy, stating: "If you have an Australian style points system and you control the quantity and quality of who comes, you know, people will sign up for that" (Chang 2016). This statement echoes the now infamous statement made by former Australian prime minister, John Howard who announced in 2001, during the election campaign that: "we will decide who comes to this country and the circumstances in which they come" (Maley 2016, p. 676). Indigenous Australians could well have echoed similar sentiments in 1788.

As in the USA against the election of Trump, there have been protests across Britain against the vote to leave the EU. Writing for the *Huffington Post,* Demianyk (2016) reports that Farage told Fox News in the USA that: "the only people resisting Brexit and a Donald Trump presidency are full-time professional protesters who didn't vote in the first place because they can't get out of bed". There are some common threads here which link the current political climates in Australia, the USA and the UK: concerns regarding the economy, immigration, the maintenance of national identity and a nostalgic return to 'greatness'. The desire for a return to the nostalgic nationalistic notion of a past greatness is not convincing. As Blackshaw (2010, p. 39) points out: "Liquid modern community today might come with its own uplifting messages, but the shame is that it is hardly ever convincing. A kind of grand narrative of community". It seems that there is also a commonality of the element of 'surprise' associated with the resurgence of the One Nation Party in Australia, Brexit in Britain and the unpredicted election of Donald Trump over seemingly 'sure thing' candidate Hilary Clinton in the USA. This state of affairs has been succinctly described by Paul Oosting, Director of Getup! Australia:[1]

> Brexit, Trump, and on our own shores, the resurgence of One Nation. There's a growing nexus between economic disadvantage and racially motivated resentment that is overwhelming all political expectations. There has been an abject failure of progressives both here and abroad to understand this, let alone counter it. And when right-wing demagogues tap this pulsing vein of resentment, we've mocked it as an ignorant fringe or dismissed it as isolated extremism.

A shift towards the political right has been building but despite its visibility, it seems that it was not taken seriously enough. In the USA, the election of Don-

---

[1]"Getup is an independent left movement to build a progressive Australia and bring participation back into our democracy." The core values of this organisation are around social justice, economic fairness and environmental sustainability: www.youtube.com/user/getupaustralia, https://wwwget up.org.au.

ald Trump confirms that a groundswell presumed, to perhaps, become reasonably popular with a disgruntled section of the community arose with enough power and numbers, to take the white house. Donald Trump was not viewed as a 'real' threat and now that it has happened there is dismay among many. In the UK, many did not think that Brexit would actually take place and a close vote was predicted at worst. Now that it has happened, many are calling for another vote. In terms of Australia, Pauline Hanson's One Nation Party is in an early re-emergence phase. However, if the likes of Trump and Brexit have managed to succeed against the majority of thought, then Hanson's potential should not be discounted. A resurgence of anti-immigration sentiment not just in Australia but also in the USA and the UK will perhaps extend to other countries and be reflected in the election of more right-wing governments. What does this mean for IMGs in Australia, or wishing to come to Australia? A growing anti-immigration position may further impact on the conditions surrounding the immigration of IMGs as well as the willingness of the Australian public and the Australian medical profession to accept them. The Australian medical profession has been noted for its self-interest and uncompetitive behaviour with some professionals feeling the need to 'protect' their turf from outsiders. The political, economic and social climate around an anti-immigration stance is already seen in the current coalition government via Australia's adoption of a tough protection of sovereign borders initiative. Clearly, there is currently a conservative political shift occurring and this is not a new phenomenon.

## What Happened?

What are the conditions necessary to bring about such a political shift? Hall (1979, p. 14) argues that: "This is a matter of a set of discontinuous but related histories, rather than neat, corresponding movements". Additionally, these histories are evasive and difficult to analyse. This may be because the left attempts to analyse from within rational, respectable and well-known positions which are now inadequate for analysis. Fundamentally, the right is what it is because the left is what it is. This presents itself as a constant class struggle. Hall (1979, p. 15) suggests:

> What shifts them is not "thoughts" but a particular practice of class struggle: ideological and political class struggle. What makes these representations popular is that they have a purchase on practice, they shape it, they are written into its materiality. What constitutes them as a danger is that they change the nature of the terrain itself on which struggles of different kinds are taking place; and they have pertinent effects on these struggles.

Communities may become disenchanted and disengage. Commenting on the 'liquid' stage of modernity and individualisation, Bauman (2013, p. 86) sheds light on community disengagement:

> The perception of injustice and of the grievances it triggers, like so much else in the times of disengagement which define the 'liquid' stage of modernity, has undergone a process of *individualisation*. Troubles are supposed to be suffered and coped with alone and are

singularly unfit for cumulation into a community of interests which seeks collective solutions to individual troubles.

Standing (2011) presents the notion of a new class, a dangerous class. The Precariat is a class in the making and constitutes a frustrated and angry socio-economic group living with insecurity and without agency. It is not yet a class-for-itself but can be likened to the proletariat or a working class (following Marx). Their precariousness, however, is being normalised in globalised labour markets and as suggested by Redhead (2015, pp. 10–11):

> We have moved, unerringly from cosmopolis to claustropolis, though, of course, never completely, and only in a roundabout way. Uneven development is always with us, as is reproletarianisation. The narrow theoretical ledge from which to view this new claustropolitanism passing by at the speed of light seems more precarious by the minute, but finding space on it is a necessary condition for survival.

The nationalist ideal therefore of countries returning to or retaining 'greatness' as espoused by Hanson, Farage and Trump is not possible. Standing (2011, p. 7) suggests: "Perhaps the reality is that we need a new vocabulary, one reflecting class relations in the global market system of the twenty-first century". The Precariat instead has a 'truncated status' in that while it has class characteristics:

> It has none of the social contract relationships of the proletariat…it also has a peculiar status position, in not mapping neatly onto high-status professional or middle-status craft occupations (Standing 2011, p. 8).

Status is often related to an individual's occupation, but this is problematic as within an occupation there can be: "divisions and hierarchies that involve very different statuses" (Standing 2011, p. 8). The positioning of IMGs within Australia's medical culture is indicative of this context. IMGs while medical professionals do not hold the same status as their Australian trained medical colleagues. The IMG community then is a separate division with lower status. It is also clear that there is a hierarchy within medicine itself: with general practitioners at the bottom and surgeons at the top and again within the surgical specialities: with general surgeons occupying the bottom position and neurosurgeons at the top.

Any worker can become a member of the Precariat due to changed circumstances or choice. Migrants, however, are particularly vulnerable, especially in wealthy countries. A central key to the right shift in politics in Australia, the USA and the UK is immigration. Migrants are demonised in public discourse; a most common concern is the belief that migrants take local jobs. The response by governments is often to enact stricter controls around migration but this global problem is more related to an evolving and growing flexible labour market rather than migrant workers. Real permanent jobs and careers are in decline while there is an increasing casualisation of the workforce. The result is a lack of job/income security leading to underemployment or unemployment. This is the case for many IMGs. Australia's immigration policies have a long history of xenophobic responses to outsiders and seem to have become more extreme over time. Hand in hand with the perception that migrants take jobs, is a kind of paranoia that Australia will be overwhelmed with a flood of migrants, refugees and asylum seekers, particularly those who come via boats. This is not the case as Maley (2016, p. 672) clearly demonstrates, arguing that: ..."even if all unauthorised boat arrivals over the last forty years were to be seated in the Melbourne Cricket Ground over a quarter of the seats would remain vacant." In fact, boat arrivals in 2013 only constituted 0.89 persons per thousand of the Australian population (Australian Bureau of Statistics 2013).

## Australia's Boat People Paranoia

Unjustified hostility towards migrants is not confined to Australia. There are growing tensions around the world. Standing (2011, p. 114) mentioned a 2009 poll conducted in the USA, UK and six countries within Europe. The UK was the most anti migrants, where 60% believed they took local jobs as compared to the USA showing 42%. Subsequent polls conducted in 2010 revealed that attitudes towards migrants had deteriorated across all the countries polled. Currently, Europe is facing a migration crisis, on a scale not seen since the Second World War. Large numbers of people are fleeing from the Middle East and Africa. In Syria, for example, where there is terrorist activity, extreme violence and infrastructure collapse, 12 million people are left in need of humanitarian aid, while 4 million people have managed to escape elsewhere (Brannan et al. 2016). Many people have no choice but to escape via boats and the most popular route from Turkey to the Greek Islands is perilous. Unfortunately, many desperate people have drowned. The ones who survive are likely to find themselves in hastily constructed, inadequate and overcrowded refugee camps in Europe. Brannan et al. (2016) while noting that the exact scale of loss of life is difficult to assess, highlight the dire situation:

> The UN High Commissioner for Refugees (UNHCR) estimates over 590,000 people have arrived in Europe by sea this year. The countries at the forefront are Greece and Italy, these countries which were never designed for such high level of migration, are inadequate.

Australia has continually implemented harsh measures to restrict and discourage boat people and the people smugglers who organise their sometimes treacherous voyages. Both the Labor Party and the Liberal Party have introduced various exclusionary policies since 1989. Labor governments in the 1990s introduced mandatory detention for boat people and repeatedly attempted to reduce their legal entitlements. Labor also initiated the Pacific and Papua New Guinea (PNG) Solutions in 2001. John Howard's Liberal–National coalition government continued in this manner particularly after the rise of Pauline Hanson's One Nation Party. In late 2007, Labor returned to power and resolved to dismantle the PNG solution but due to an increase in boat arrivals, reintroduced it in 2013.

Throughout the 2000s, as Glynn (2016, p. 3) notes:

> Australia drew on its economic advantages to tempt various Pacific island nations, and more recently Cambodia, to house and resettle boat people in exchange for valuable aid and investment.

The Cambodian attempt was outrageously expensive and unsuccessful. In his opinion piece, Riley (2016) reports: "The government spent $55 million to transfer five refugees to Cambodia. Only two remained for any length of time, and the Cambodian government admitted that its government "does not have the social programs to support them". The current 'solution' (to what exactly, I am not entirely sure) in Australia, is Operation Sovereign Borders. This title is not surprising, however, as immigration overall is handled by the Department of Immigration and Border Protection. However, from 2007 until September 2013 the responsible department was called The Department of Immigration and Citizenship which was preceded by the Department of Immigration and Multicultural Affairs. Perhaps the departmental name changes indicate a shift in Australia's stance regarding immigration, from suspicion and caution to a paranoidal focus on exclusion to facilitate protection. To protect Australia, our response to boat people is to make sure they do not set foot on Australian soil. Numerous discriminatory legislations have been introduced by various governments over time, the following is just one example from 2001 outlined by Glynn (2016, pp. 128–129):

> one privative clause was designed to ensure that a decision to reject an asylum seeker's application for refugee status could not 'be challenged, appealed against, reviewed, quashed or called in question in any court'. This followed several previous Australian governments' ineffective attempts to reduce the influence of NGOs and lawyers representing asylum seekers. In Ruddock's[2] words, this hard-line political response would ensure that 'unauthorised arrivals do not achieve their goal of reaching Australian soil; there is no automatic access to Australian residency; [and,] there is no access to the judicial system.

Until recently, Australia was sending asylum seekers to Manus Island in PNG and the Pacific island of Nauru. According to operation sovereign borders, in September 2016 there were 873 asylum seekers on Manus Island and 396 on Nauru (Australian Government Department of Immigration and Border Protection 2016). Government policy, according to Riley (2016), is based on disproportionate fear, in that if the government reconsiders and agrees to resettle asylum seekers in Australia people smuggling via boat will escalate. Riley (2016) argues that:

> this is very unlikely. Given the manifest immediate harm to refugees and asylum seekers on Nauru and Manus Island, it is worth risking the resumption of boat arrivals to solve the humanitarian crisis on our doorstep that is entirely of Australia's making.

The government's rationale and the rhetoric around its border protection approach have been the demonisation of people smugglers and the responsibility to do our humanitarian best by discouraging them. A tough stance was espoused as a life-saving initiative which would ultimately prevent the drowning of boat people trying to reach Australia. In a joint press conference (Miller 2016) with Peter Dutton then minister for Immigration and Border Protection, prime minister Turnbull stated that the government was locked in: a "battle of wills with criminal gangs of people smugglers. You should not underestimate the scale of the threat. These people smugglers are the worst criminals imaginable". The latest policy initiative proposed in October

---

[2]Phillip Ruddock was Australia's Attorney General in 2001.

2016 is the strongest most exclusionary initiative to-date. The government announced that any asylum seekers including all those detained on Manus Island and Nauru at any time since the last half of 2013 will never be accepted to enter Australia on temporary or permanent visas (including tourist visas). The reality of this announcement will result in family trauma, as noted by Riley (2016):

> This will prevent asylum seekers who have family in Australia from ever meeting them in Australia. We know anecdotally that there are asylum seekers and refugees on Nauru and Manus Island in this position. Indeed, it is common for refugees to follow the same path to protection as family members who had earlier fled persecution.

In addition, this will prevent asylum seekers from perhaps re-entering Australia years after their detention to undertake studies or to conduct business. The impetus for this policy again is based on a xenophobic fear that somehow asylum seekers denied access will return from a country where they have been resettled and try again. Minister Dutton in Tom McIlroy's article in *The Age* (2016) is quoted:

> What we don't want is if someone is to go to a third country, that they apply for a tourist visa or some other way to circumvent what the government's policy intent is by coming back to Australia from that third country.

Boat arrivals since 1998 have increasingly been depicted as some kind of 'national emergency'. Firstly, asylum seekers coming via boat have been portrayed as illegal 'queue jumpers'. Maley (2016, p. 673) argues:

> This is an entirely spurious claim: it is not an offence under any Australian law to seek to enter the country without a visa and internationally there is no 'queue' for refugees to 'jump', given that resettlement programmes do not offer a place in a queue but a ticket in a lottery.

This term and the rhetoric around it, while created by bureaucrats, managed to gain significant support from the general public. Maley (2016, p. 674) places the stance into perspective and maintains that:

> This is once again a suspect line of argument at multiple levels. It has overtones of the 'whiteman's burden': that the kind of people who board boats could not possibly be capable of thinking for themselves, and therefore need others to do their thinking for them. It does not explain why causes of mortality such as the road toll, which routinely produces more than 1000 deaths a year in Australia, have led to virtually no public emoting by political leaders.

If Australia was to act genuinely humanely, it would consider the source causes of refugee movements and realise that if the route to Australia is a 'closed' one, then this forces people to find another route, perhaps one that is even more dangerous than the route by sea to Australia (Donini et al. 2016). Perhaps Australians are not really concerned for the safety of refugees, preferring not to welcome refugees at all.

For example, what one chooses to wear is a covert way of displaying opinion or making a statement. I first saw a t-shirt featuring a map of Australia with the words F*** OFF WE'RE FULL[3] on the front in a local supermarket. I was shocked.

---

[3]"Show your Aussie Pride with this classic t-shirt design. Made of 100% cotton, this shirt would make the perfect Christmas gift for the patriotic Australian in your household". AUD $22.70 accessed 14/12/2016 https://teespring.com/shop/australiana#pid=2&cid=2397&sid=front.

Overtly xenophobic and racist, seemingly unafraid of possible reaction, it was worn by a middle-aged man who went about his shopping. Unfortunately, I saw this same t-shirt several times on different individuals (all males) on different occasions. Through its persistent anti-asylum seeker/refugee rhetoric, the government has been able to influence the thoughts of many Australian citizens and now with the current approach has sent a very clear message to the world. Riley (2016) sums up the message:

> The government's message to people who might subsequently attempt to get to Australia is loud and clear: you are not welcome, you will not be resettled in Australia, you will spend many years in remote locations that will lead many of you to develop serious mental illness, and many of you will commit suicide or self-harm. We cannot guarantee your safety at these locations. You risk being murdered or sexually assaulted. Things will be so bad that many of you will choose to return to your country of origin, where you fear persecution, rather than tolerate these conditions.

It is clear that Australia does not readily welcome the 'other' and is a xenophobic, fearful nation. Immigration, however, has been central in the Australian population from the nineteenth century and a part of the ideal of a white Australian nation populated with British people. Although, small numbers of other Europeans were tolerated on the basis that they would assimilate into the mainstream population, however: "coloured immigration was almost completely excluded" (Carter 2006, p. 329). After the Second World War, the mass immigration program to boost the population increased the pool of potential migrants and this began to transform the ethnic and cultural composition of Australia. By the 1970s, the result was a change in immigration policy and therefore a transformation of Australia as now a 'multicultural' nation.

However, increased levels of immigrants from Asia in the 1970s and 1980s brought about fresh fears of change and particularly a perceived threat to stability and social cohesion. Carter (2006, p. 329) concludes:

> It is clear that large-scale immigration has had profound social and cultural effects on Australian society. The voices of anxiety and reaction are responding to real social change, both in Australia and globally (as are the advocates of ever larger immigration intakes). ...racial categories remain powerful in mainstream conceptions of the Australian nation, no less so for no longer being named or understood as racial.

The asylum seekers of today are the scapegoats for a renewed and backdated vigour of government attention and punishment. The extent to which the current Australian government will go in its excessive nationalist quest in the recent push to further alienate asylum seekers and refugees from Australia beggars belief. My sentiments are aligned with Riley's (2016, p. 6):

> Since October 2013, nearly 2500 asylum seekers have had to suffer for the Australian government to send this message. Does it really need to add to the list of detriments that asylum seekers will never enter Australia in any capacity for the rest of their lives? Where does it end?

This is the Australian nation IMGs come to, the nation they wish to live and work in, sharing their much needed professional skills. For IMGs, this is an Australia that sends very mixed messages, one that this country represents an egalitarian society with a 'fair go' for all as opposed to one that marginalizes and excludes certain groups of people who are othered (Plage et al. 2016). The Australian nation and its nationalist stance are clearly an intersecting oppression for IMGs. Intertwined with nation is race which has been at the heart of the country since the 1788 invasion by the British. The creation of the 'new' Australian nation required the dispossession of Australia's Indigenous peoples, and they were systematically excluded. Vehicles for exclusion included their physical confinement to reserves and missions. They were assigned a separate and inferior legal status and cultural and psychological exclusion (Reid et al. 2016). "This exclusion was through, an extraordinary forgetfulness, a voluntary amnesia which rendered them invisible within the nation" (Stanner 1969). Racism towards Indigenous Australians is still very much embedded and institutionalized within the structure of society and in the minds of many Australians. For example, the journal reflection made by a Bachelor of Education student in Merridy Malin's (1997, p. 49) study of an Anti-Racism Teacher Education Program. The student's reflection concludes with:

> Where would the Aboriginal be now if the British didn't settle here? They wouldn't be as well off as they are now would they? Sure they would have the land but nothing else. No money, alcohol, cars and tobacco just to name a few. They would have none of this.

Another example, in a similar vein, was published online in 2000. It was circulated by students at several universities in Australia (including the one at which I was employed) in 2002.

Entitled "Australian Apology to the Aboriginals", it lists several 'apologies' including:

> We feel that we must apologise for building hundreds of homes for you, which you have vandalised and destroyed. We apologise for giving you doctors and free medical care which allowed you to survive and multiply so that you can demand apologies. We apologise for giving you law and order, which has helped prevent you from slaughtering one another. We humbly beg your forgiveness for all these sins and are happy to take back all the above and return you to the paradise of the outback whenever you are ready.[4]

Many Australians openly express racist, xenophobic and ethnocentric views but insist that those views are not. One notable example came from an Australian prime minister. In 1997, the Howard government was presented with the Bringing Them Home Report (Human Rights and Equal Opportunities Commission 1997). The report detailed many oral histories of Indigenous Australians who were forcibly removed from their families as children (often referred to as the Stolen Generations). The report recommended that Australian governments publicly apologise for the past harmful policies. The response of the Howard government was to reject and dispute the report. In fact, the past practices by governments was defended and justified by the Howard government as 'doing the right thing'. Hocking (2010, p. 57) describes the feeling at the time:

---

[4]The full 'apology' can be accessed at Australia's e-journal of social and political debate (Post and Reposte by Tim Dunlop 19 April 2000) http://onlineopinion.com.au?view.asp?article=107g page = 2.

This attitude fed the racism of many Australians who agreed with John Howard. Without even perhaps reading at least one of the oral histories contained in the report or perhaps without any understanding of the racist policy which led to this particular part of our shared history.

It was not until February 2008 that a national apology was made by the newly elected Labor prime minister, Kevin Rudd. Moreover, in 2009, the Rudd government finally endorsed the United Nations Declaration on the Rights of Indigenous Peoples. Until this time, Australia was opposed to the declaration and abstained from voting. The previous Howard government failed to sincerely recognise the rights of Australia's Indigenous peoples, much of this stance was based on fear. The government and wider community feared that perhaps Traditional law could challenge National law and clear the way for Indigenous Australians to make claims.

## We're Not Racists! But...

The Australian national ideology is founded on 'whiteness', obtaining it, keeping it and perpetuating it. In fact, the first legislation to come from the new Federation Parliament in 1901 led to the White Australia Policy, which was in place until the 1960s (Hirst 2014). Ironically, the country was full of black Australians, another marker of the invisibility of Indigenous Australians, and also a chosen ignorance to the invisibility of a social reality. Colour can in fact bring a hypervisibility to certain groups. Eloquently explained by Sefa Dei (2008, p. 83):

> Social identities morph into complex configurations. Through time human societies have morphed into configurations. Identities are historically contingent and specific...While identities are fluid, we must also recognise the "permanence" – as in its longstanding evocation – of skin colour as a salient marker of identity through time, history and space. It is in this understanding that we herald the power of race in intersectional analyses...the significance of colour in the mind of the racist cannot be dismissed.

The white/black binary opposition has ancient roots. 'Blackness' and 'whiteness' are embedded in medieval European christian texts, for example. Whiteness was seen as an important part of christian identity, a colour of salvation and goodness while blackness was the colour of hell and evil (Ken 2008). Whiteness is more than identity. Following Frankenberg (1993), whiteness is discourse, structure and location. Power and privilege play a central role in how whiteness works. Colour and racial/ethnic origins can be applied to whites and blacks. The difference is that for blacks the application has resulted in profound outcomes of loss, whereas for whites it has meant privilege. In addition, privilege for the West. As Moreton-Robinson an Indigenous academic explains (2004, p. 75):

> Because in the West whiteness defines itself as the norm...in this way whiteness is constitutive of the epistemology of the West; it is an invisible regime of power that secures hegemony through discourse and has material effects in everyday life.

Indigenous disadvantage in Australia has become in itself a wicked problem, as despite numerous efforts by governments to be seen to be 'doing something' disadvantage has not been addressed. I would argue that this is because governments are not willing to hand over real power and opportunity to Indigenous communities, particularly full, equal access to the economy. Moreover, the Australian nation would not allow governments to do so. At the core here is racism, an ethnocentric white supremacy and xenophobia fuelled by entrenched negative stereotypes and ideological/political baggage. In terms of IMGs in Australia, those with dark skin can be viewed as carrying a double burden or layer of difference; firstly, because they belong to an underclass within the medical profession and secondly because they are black. During conversations with interview participants in this study, some shared perceptions of a black/white binary lived experience. In our interview, when I asked Colin (2010, Interview 2) how his wife had settled into Australia, he expressed concern for her loneliness. Colin's wife was a high school teacher but her qualifications were not accepted in Australia. Colin stated: "people here won't talk to her". I asked him why he thought that was the case, and he replied: "because she is black skinned I suppose". Shaun (2012, Interview 8) considered himself, in some ways, fortunate: "Well, I have an accent but at least I'm not black". Whereas, Gary (2012, Interview 9) considered himself more fortunate, and stated with a knowing smile: "I don't have black skin and not a really strong accent, so I go under that radar. I think my patients get surprised when they ask me where I'm from".

This leads to a questioning of identity, and in terms of the IMG community particularly, professional identity. IMGs come to Australia with the professional identity of medical doctor but almost immediately, the processes and discourses of the system begin to erode that identity, constantly calling it into question.

## IMGs and Professional Identity

The intersecting expressions of class, race and nation in the representation of IMG experience in Australia impact on their professional and personal identity. Intersectionality aims to connect identity with other forms of difference. Sefa Dei (2008, p. 85) argues:

> Critical anti-racist work, whether pursued as part of intersectional or interlocking analyses, calls for subverting the dominance meanings (meta-narratives) surrounding the use of…-categories. We do so by recognising the distinction between the 'metaphor' and the 'real' and how, for some bodies, the permanence of these categories are refracted in the daily experiences.

In their fascinating research into the use of space by medically unemployed IMGs in Victorian hospitals, Harris and Guillemin (2015) reveal an adaptive culture which has evolved out of need and agency. A kind of medical underground for IMGs exists in the margins outside of clinical activity but within the hospital environment. These IMGs as a professional community try to keep their identity as medical doctors while striving to study for registration assessments and have contact with other IMG community members. The most popular "congregational nodes" within the hospital were usually, the library, cafeteria and tutorial room. The scene is poignantly described (Harris and Guillemin 2015, p. 168):

> Amongst the textbooks and teaching models, the IMGs had a heightened sense of medical identity. Alongside other IMGs, they could try to survive the tediousness of study and efface the loneliness of life in textbooks. At the same time the skeletons and anatomical dummies with their organs fitting neatly together, the ordered filing systems and carefully delineated places and times of study, reiterated forms of control; these paralleled the regulating principles of the registration process the IMGs were enmeshed in, the place mirroring their position in the hierarchy. IMGs were delineated in this place from the staff 'with passes'; they were grouped with students, also on the medical periphery, and allowed access only to distinguished areas at designated times.

The hospital was symbolic of a medical identity for IMGs, a connection to their study days as medical students and while perhaps a source of empowerment in terms of solidarity as a community, very much reflecting back to them their status, as an underclass within Australia's medical culture.

The intersecting oppressions of inequality: class, race and nation all conspire to subjugate IMGs to an underclass within Australia's medical culture. This book moves towards an explanation of why IMGs are positioned as such. The Australian nation has a long history of xenophobia where the other is viewed not only with suspicion and fear but as inferior. Racism also lurks in every fibre of the growth of the 'new' nation from 1788 to today. It is evidenced by the adoption of the White Australia Policy in 1901 to the current chronic failure of governments to address Indigenous Australian disadvantage. Whiteness is the epistemology of Western democracies and the associated norms, values and beliefs have been enshrined in laws rendering exclusionary ideas and actions institutionalised into Australian society and into the structures and operations of Australian institutions. Hence, it follows that the various bodies constructed to regulate and manage IMGs and their entry into medical practice in Australia reek of and reflect: class, race and nation. IMGs find themselves positioned within these disempowering oppressive intersections which are interconnected and fluid. This chapter has explored the paradigm of intersectionality and its potential to confront inequitable power relations. Australia's immigration policies have been exposed as exclusionary and inhumane. They are underpinned by Australia's obsession for whiteness and fear of the foreign other, xenophobia. The government has succeeded in demonising those who are the most vulnerable and needy who try to come to our shores. There is a Western world political shift as seen in the rise of the One Nation Party in Australia as well as the election of Donald Trump to the US presidency and the UK vote to leave the EU (Brexit). These results represent an angry working-class backlash often seen in ailing economies with high unemployment. This political phenomenon has been explored for common concerns, that of perceived job loss due to immigration and the resurgence of nationalism. As a result, these political times also represent a concern for IMGs and global medical migration.

The following concluding discussion brings together themes and thoughts. The future and what it could look like is also advanced, but it is the future that always holds some mysteries and surprises and I am sure Medicine in Australia will be no exception.

# References

Armstrong, P., & Britton, B. (2016). Nigel Farage: Arch-eurosceptic and brexit "puppet master". *CNN*. Viewed November 15, 2016. http://edition.cnn.com/2016/06/24/europe/eu-referendum-ni gel-farage/index.html.

Australian Bureau of Statistics. (2013). *Australian demographic statistics: March 2013*. Australian Bureau of Statistics, viewed November 12, 2016. http://www.abs.gov.au/AUSSTATS/abs@nsf/Lookup/3101.0.

Australian Government Department of Immigration and Border Protection. (2016). Australian Government. Viewed October 5, 2016. https://www.border.gov.au.

Bacchi, C. (2009). *Analysing policy: What's the problem represented to be?*. Frenchs Forest, NSW: Pearson Australia.

Bauman, Z. (Ed.). (2013). *Community: Seeking safety in an insecure world*, Wiley. Viewed April 10, 2017, (ProQuest Ebook Central). http://ebookcentral.proquest.com.ezproxy.flinders.edu.au/l ib/flinders/detail.action?docID=1187719.

Blackshaw, T. (2010). *Key concepts in community studies*. Sage key concepts series London: Sage Publications.

Brannan, S., Campbell, R., Davies, M., English, V., Mussell, R. & Sheather, J. C. (2016). The Mediterranean refugee crisis: Ethics, international law and migrant health. *Journal of Medical Ethics*, *42*(4), 269–270.

Brown, L., & Strega, S. (2005). *Research as resistance: Critical, indigenous and anti-oppressive approaches*. Toronto: Canadian Scholars' Press.

Carter, D. (2006). *Dispossession, dreams & diversity: Issues in Australian studies*. Frenchs Forest, NSW: Pearson Educatiion Australia.

Chang, C. (2016). Who is UKIP leader Nigel Farage? *news.com.au*. Viewed November 15, 2016. http://www.news.com.au/world/europe/who-is-ukip-leader-nigel-farage/news-story/3e5f1 ccef6c2b03b91aadc8eb6c6d9eb.

Choo, H. Y., & Ferree, M. M. (2010). Practicing intersectionality in sociological research. *Sociological Theory, 28*(2), 129–49.

Crenshaw, K. (1989). Demarginalizating the intersection of race and sex: A black feminist critique of antidiscrimination doctorine, feminist theory, and antiracist politics. *University of Chicago Legal Forum, 14,* 538–554.

Eckermann, A. K., Dowd, T., Chong, E., Nixon, L., Gray, R., & Johnson, S. (2006). *Binan Goonj: Bridging cultures in Aboriginal health* (2nd ed.). Marrickville: Churchill Livingstone Elsevier.

Fraser, H. & Taylor, N. (2016). *Species, gender and class and the production of knowledge*. Palgrave Macmillan, (Flinders university) http://www.springer.com/series/14707.

Demianyk, G. (2016). Nigel Farage dismisses anti-donald trump and brexit protestors as 'professionals' too lazy to vote. *The huffington post*. Viewed November 14, 2016. http://www.huffingto npost.co.uk/entry/nigel-farage-donald-trump-protests_uk_5828921de4b09ac74c528c04.

Donini, A., Monsutti, A., & Scalettaris, G. (2016). *Afgans on the move: Seeking protection and refuge in Europe. In this journey I died several times; in Afghanisstan you only die once*, Geneva.

Ernst, J. (2016). After Trump, a call for political correctness from the right. *Right Press*. Viewed November 14, 2016. http://us.pressfrom.com/news/opinion/-4164-after-trump-a-call-for-politic al-correctness-from-the-right/.

Frankenberg, R. (1993). *White women, race matters: The social construction of whiteness*. Routledge, London & New York.

Foucault, M. (1972). *The Archaeology of knowledge*. Tavistock, London.

Galtung, J. (1970). Feudal systems, structural violence and the structural theory of revolution. *Revista Latinoamericana de Ciencia Politica, 1*(1), 25–79.

Galtung, J. (1990). Cultural violence. *Journal of Peace Research, 27*, 291–305, viewed May 16, 2012. http://jpr.sagepub.com/.

Glynn, I. (2016). *Asylum policy, boat people and political discourse: Boats, votes and asylum in Australia and Italy*. Palgrave Macmillan, UK. Viewed November 8, 2016, via Springer link (Flinders university). http://download.springer.com.exyproxy.

Hall, S. (1979). The great moving right show. *Marxism today*.

Harris, A., & Guillemin, M. (2015). Notes on the medical underground: Migrant doctors at the margins. *Health Sociology Review, 24*(2), 163–174. Viewed March 21, 2016. http://dx.doi.org/1 0.1080/14461242.2014.999403.

Hill Collins, P. (1990). *Black feminist thought: Knowledge, consciousness, and the politics of empowerment* (Vol. 2)., Perspectives on gender Boston: Unwin Hyman.

Hill Collins, P. (2000). *Black feminist thought: Knowledge consciousness, and the politics of empowerment* (2nd ed.). New York: Routledge.

Hill Collins, P. (2010). The new politics of community. *American Sociological Review, 75*(1), 7–30. Viewed September 6, 2012. https://doi.org/10.1177/0003122410363293. Via Sage (downloaded from www.asr.sagepub.com at Adelaide theological library) http://asr.sagepub.com.

Hill Collins, P., & Bilge, S. (2016). *Intersectionality*. Cambridge, UK: Polity press.

Hirst. (2014). *Australian history in 7 questions*. Black Inc., Collingwood Vic.

Hocking, D. (2010). Sorry seemed to be the hardest word. In A. Gunstone (Ed.), *Over a decade of despair: The howard government and indigenous affairs* (pp. 51–74). Australian Scholarly Publishing Pty. Ltd., North Melbourne.

Human Rights and Equal Opportunities Commission. (1997). *Bringing them home: Report of the National Inquiry into the separation of Aboriginal and Torres Strait Islander children from their families*. Sydney.

Ken, I. (2008). Beyond the intersection: A new culinary metaphor for race-class-gender studies. *Sociological Theory, 26*, 152–721. Viewed January 23, 2014, via Sage Publications (Flinders University) stx.sagepub.com.

Le Messurier, D. (2016). One nation senator Pauline Hanson makes toasts to Donald Trump victory. Viewed November 11, 2016. http://www.news.com.au/nationalpolitics/one-nation-senator-pauli ne-hanson-makes-toasts-donald-trump-to-victory/news/story.

Lutz, H., Herrera Vivar, M. T., & Supik, L. (Eds.). (2011). *Framing intersectionality: Debates on multi-faceted concept in gender studies*. Surrey: Ashgate Publishing.

Maley, W. (2016). Australia's refugee policy: Domestic politics and diplomatic consequences. *Australian Journal of International Affairs, 70*(6), 670–680. Viewed November 8, 2016. Via Routledge taylor and francis group (Flinders University). http://www.tandfonline.com.exproxy.

Malin, M. (1997). An anti-racism teacher education program. In S. Harris & M. Malin (Eds.), *Indigenous education: Historical, moral and practical tales*. Northern Territory University Press, Darwin.

McIlroy, T. (2016). Immigration minister Peter Dutton says new refugee ban will stop country hopping. *The Age*. Viewed November 21, 2016. http://www.theage.cpm.au/federal-politics-ne ws/immigration-minister-peter-dutton-says-new-refugee-ban-will-stop-country-hopping-20161 030-gse8jx.html.

Miller, P. (2016). Australian Associated Press. *Press conference Dutton and Turnbull*. ABC News. Viewed November 7, 2016, https://www.abc.net.au/news/2016-11-05/peter-dutton-malcolm-tur nbull-immigration-press-conference/7997154.

Moreton-Robinson, A. (2004). Whiteness, epistemology and indigenous representation. In A. Moreton-Robinson (Ed.), *Whitening race: Essays in social and cultural criticism* (pp. 75–88). Canberra: Aboriginal studies press for the AIATSIS.

Museum Victoria. (1996). Viewed November 12, 2016. https://wwwmuseumvictoria.com.au.

One Nation Party. (2016). Viewed November 11, 2016. http://www.onenation.com.au.

Plage, S., Willing, I., Skrbis, Z., & Woodward, I. (2016). Australiannes as fairness: Implications for cosmopolitan encounters. *Journal of Sociology, 1*(6), 1–16, viewed February 9, 2017, via Sage (Flinders University, South Australia) http://jos.sagepub.com.

Phillips, T. (2016). China threatens to cut sales of i.phones and US cars if 'naive' Trump pursues trade war. *The Guardian.* Viewed November 15, 2016. http://www.theguardian.com/world/2016/nov/14/china-threatens-to-cut-sales-of-i.phones-and-us-cars-if-naive-trump-pursues-trade-war.

Poliplatform. (2016). *Donald Trump's policies.* Viewed November 14, 2016. https://www.donaldtrump'spoliciespolitiplatform.com/trump.

Redhead, S. (2015). *Football and accelerated culture: This modern sporting life.*, Routledge research in sport, culture and society London: Routledge Taylor & Francis Group.

Reid, J. S., Taylor, K., & Hayes, C. (2016). Indigenous health systems and services. In E. Willis, L. Reynolds & H. Keleher (Eds.), *Understanding the Australian health care system* (pp. 153–66). Elsevier Chatswood.

Riley, A. (2016). Same old rhetoric cannot justify banning refugees from Australia. *The Conversation.* Viewed November 17, 2016. http://www.theconversation.com/same-old-rhetoric-cannot-justify-banning-refugees-from-australia-67923.

Savitch, H. V. (1975). The politics of deprivation. In H. R. Rogers & W. A. Freeman (Eds.), *Racism and inequality: The policy alternatives* (pp. 5–36). San Fransisco.

Sefa Dei, G. J. (2008). Race, difference, and the discourse of intersectionality. *Racists beware: Uncovering racial politics in the post modern society* (pp. 81–91). The Netherlands: Sense publishers.

Standing, G. (2011). *The Precariat: The new dangerous class.* London: Bloomsbury Academic.

Stanner, W. E. H. (1969). *After the dreaming. Black and white Australians: An anthropologist's view.* Sydney.

Sydney Morning Herald. (2016). Viewed November 12, 2016. http://wwwsmh.com.au/federalpolitics/political-news/pauline-hansons-2016-maiden-speech-to-the-senate-fulltranscript-20160.

White, R. (1997). Inventing Australia revisited. In W. Hudson & G. Bolton (Eds.), *Creating Australia: Changing Australian history.* Allen & Unwin, Sydney.

Willis, E. (1989). *Medical dominance: The division of labour in Australian health care* (revised ed.). Allen & Unwin, North Sydney.

# Conclusion: Where to from Here? Transformation or a Very Wicked Problem

I know that a number of them feel like they think they are perceived as second-class in the system and there are plenty of Australian doctors that will talk with them in those terms. I think that is a sad thing and we are going to end up with a very fragmented profession out there. Some of the doctors who have come to Australia have been specialists from where they have come from and have academic work behind them and would have to have been highly regarded in their country of origin, very established. I can think of people who have done a lot of academic work in South Africa and come here and are treated as if they would barely rate to qualify for the profession. I know that for a number of them that is a very difficult thing and they really resent the number of hurdles put in front of them. It insults their intelligence and their pride. The fact that they have to go back and prove themselves so much and even when they do still not be accepted, that is a major factor that we see quite a bit. They come back at me and say, 'Why do we need to do this?' Some of them accept it and some don't. It is a difficulty for them, yet if you are a UK trained graduate you will be accepted straight in as if you were on an equal basis. (Informant in Hawthorne et al. 2004, p. 67)

The emphasis on consumerism and managerialism has legitimized and advanced the individual pursuit of material self-interest and the standardization of professional work which are the very vices for which professions have been criticized, preserving form without spirit. (Freidson 2001, p. 181)

This book is essentially underpinned by an exploration of the power structures which infiltrate the experiences of IMGs in Australia. Analysis has not produced a 'truth': rather this study has searched for the processes which assign 'truth' to some forms of discourse above other forms of discourse. Power struggles however can be the source of transformation. Drawing on the work of Hook (2001), Macias (2015, p. 238) in her discussion on Foucault's work points out:

Illuminating moments in which power struggles determine how discourse evolves normative discourses experience moments of weakness, uncertainty, and rearticulation present important transformative possibilities, because it is in these moments that we see that things do not have to be the way they are.

Foucault stressed the need to develop a sceptical attitude and a critical understanding of power and how it works as well as a need to: "know how, and to what

© Springer Nature Singapore Pte Ltd. 2019
V. A. Pascoe, *Australia's Toxic Medical Culture*,
https://doi.org/10.1007/978-981-13-2426-0_8

extent, it might be possible to think differently, instead of legitimating what is already known" (Foucault 1985, p. 9). It appears, however, that not enough is known about the medical profession, aspects of how it operates and perhaps how to transform it. Decades of inquiries and subsequent recommendations have not addressed many fundamental and concerning issues.

The Senate Community Affairs References Committee (2016, p. 66) Recommendation 6 4.37 proposes that another new inquiry be established. This time, the suggested terms of reference for further inquiry are focussed on aspects of the National Law and whether or not changes are needed to adequately deal with medical complaints. The impetus for this recommendation has obviously been driven by the surge of complaints linked to bullying and sexual harassment within the medical profession. It is also evident that there is concern for perhaps unlawful or inadequate legal processes and patient safety, which in itself, has legal implications. Also of concern is the impact that bullying and harassment may have on patient safety. The Senate Committee (2016, p. 33) noted that:

> Bullying and harassment, identified as a prevalent issue in the medical profession, is not currently considered to have a substantial impact on patient safety. The committee is of the view that the entire medical profession needs to, as a matter of priority, recognise this significant impact.

The Health Care Consumers' Association (HCCA) (2016, submission 16, p. 11) drew the committee's attention to research which shows increasing clear evidence that medical workplaces where bullying and harassment are present also represent unsafe places for patients. The HCCA referred to current research from the USA:

> Intimidating and disruptive behaviours can foster medical errors, contribute to poor patient satisfaction and to preventable adverse outcomes, increase the cost of care, and cause qualified clinicians, administrators and managers to seek new positions in more professional environments.

Within the medical profession, there is general recognition that bullying and harassment are a significant problem. For example, the AMA (2016, submission 9, p. 1) sums up succinctly the contributing factors to the current culture within medicine:

> The hierarchical nature of medicine, gender and cultural stereotypes, power imbalance inherent in medical training, and the competitive nature of practice and training has engendered a culture of bullying and harassment that has, over time, become pervasive and institutionalised in some areas of medicine.

This state of affairs is certainly indicated by other inquiries, the voices from this study, complaints and media coverage. How many inquiries are necessary to establish that the entire profession, from the training of medical students within universities and on placement (referred to in submission 10, 2016 as a "pedagogy of humiliation"), to the questionable practice of some high-ranking senior surgeons, requires an extensive shakeup? Ward and Outram (2016, p. 112) call for collective change to develop a culture: "where sustainable medical careers can develop and better serve the community". How much change do inquiries actually instigate?

Sometimes the results of inquiry recommendations manifest in changes but are they helpful or far reaching enough? In her journal article, IMG Douglas (2008, p. 36) argues that: "In some ways the attempt to establish fairer and more flexible accreditation and registration standards for IMGs will make the situation even more complex". It has been established that the accreditation and registration processes required of IMGs are already overly complex, such as the 2012 Parliamentary Inquiry Report which likened the processes to a "bowl of spaghetti" (2012, p. 6). The question of whether or not Royal Commissions, inquiries and the like constitute truly beneficial change agents is not a new one. Burton and Carlen (1979, p. 7) critique the history of inquiries and official discourse around law and order maintaining that in the nineteenth-century inquiries often arose in response to social crisis. In contemporary society, however, with the rise of capitalism, the importance of inquiries has declined:

> They can be seen as tactical devices to defray government activity, to postpone legisla-
> tive or other action while simultaneously demonstrating that particular problems are under
> administrative review and control...moreover the recommendations of a report (when not
> 'white-washes'), being advisory, can be and frequently are ignored.

Inquiries take time and, as a result, have the potential to soothe the public and issues of concern while waiting for subsequent reports. This, in turn, can temporarily alleviate the pressure on governments and stall a response. For example, the government has yet to respond to the 2012 Inquiry report: "Lost in the Labyrinth". It must be disheartening for those IMGs who made submissions to the inquiry to be still waiting for a response, perhaps there will be no response.

It is argued here that the power of the medical profession, which gives it medical dominance status, is flawed. The weaknesses exposed within medicine, and its well-established toxic culture, have accelerated to the extent that power has failed, and medicine is imploding from within. The exploration here has extended beyond the explanation of 'how' medical dominance is created, perpetuated and retained (see Willis 1989, 2006) to the explanation of 'why' medical dominance is created, perpetuated and retained. The 'why' has played a fundamental part in discussion construction, it was the 'why' that led me to continually question and search for the reasons, interests and agendas which underpin and explain the positioning of IMGs.

As explained in the introduction, this book was initially inspired by the Dr. Patel tragedy of 2005 at the Bundaberg hospital in Queensland. This incident triggered what Dr. Haikerwal (a past president of the AMA) called: "Medical Racism" (Haikerwal 2005). Acutely aware of racism in this country, I was intrigued by its insidious ability to lurk covertly under the surface of society always present always threatening, but silent. Then, an incident or turn of events releases the beast and it erupts overtly to the surface in all its ugliness. Other IMGs also began to experience a public backlash and a 'panic' ensued calling into question the equivalence of IMG medical qualifications to those of Australian trained doctors. The government was of course expected to respond to these concerns as were the medical bureaucracy, and as a result, there was a renewed, more intense focus on the qualifications, assessment and recruitment procedures of overseas trained medical professionals entering Australia. Australia's long history of xenophobia also came to the surface to fuel the fire with suspicion of the 'other'. The rhetoric of: we must maintain Australia's high standards of healthcare delivery became the dominant discourse. The partner of racism and xenophobia, ethnocentricism joined in and superiority (underpinned by whiteness) completed the package. Subsequently, the response implied that Australian trained medical doctors were superior, because the standard of their training is among the best in the world. The health care available in Australia is second to none. Therefore, to maintain that high standard we must stringently screen medical doctors from overseas because they are foreign and their qualifications are inferior to Australian qualifications. Dr. Patel came to Australia from working in the USA. The reaction to his malpractice in Australia was one of the alarms that this medical practitioner's credentials and record of practice in the USA were not sufficiently and thoroughly checked, enabling him to secure employment and practice in Australia. In this climate, my journey began and I sought out IMG voices to gain a sense of how they might be feeling, how they experience Australia, what might be the challenges and rewards of medical practice in a new country.

A social justice, anti-oppressive stance was the best approach to take in this qualitative research study as I sought to interpret the meaning of the social reality and lived experience of IMGs as a professional community. I realised from my field work prior to data collection that the system played a part in the IMG experience but I did not realise how all encompassing and powerful the system was until the voices began to show me. I have described the system as the elephant in the room. Once its enormity and power was exposed, its presence invaded the research space and seemed to be connected in some way to every aspect of the construction of IMG lived experience. The focus group participants, the interview participants and those IMGs and others who participated through submissions to the 2012 Parliamentary Inquiry and to the 2016 Senate Community Affairs References Committee provided me with a rich data set. The culture within medicine itself has been put under the microscope. I have found the stories, at times confronting, shocking and many reveal serious violation of human rights. The highly respected elite and powerful profession of medicine is rife with bullying and sexual harassment (Sherden and Cannane 2015). The surgical fields were identified as the most septic with outrageous examples of lying, fraud, bullying and victimisation towards others to guard self-interest and market share. The extent to which some surgeons were prepared to go was criminal such as the virtual running out of town of the, by then, suicidal French surgeon Dr. Richard Emery who was the victim of false complaints and sham audits (Cannane 2015). Then, there was Neurosurgeon, Dr. Charlie Teo's revelation that surgical colleagues (guarding their reputations) were not performing operations they should, sometimes resulting in loss of life, and were reluctant to disagree with another colleague's opinion (Australian Broadcasting Commission 2016). It seemed that my journey to explore the experiences of IMGs had morphed into a Pandora's Box. The experiences highlighted a problematic relationship with the health system and with Australian trained doctors. In addition, the medical profession itself was problematic.

A social justice research agenda was adopted to maximise representation of the voices while exposing the power structures which oppress them. Intersectionality offered an emancipatory, anti-oppressive analytic tool for the exploration of intersecting social phenomena (Hill Collins and Bilge 2016) and was therefore the best way to organise and explain the experiences of IMGs in Australia. Theories around social justice explore both social reality and the possibility for social justice (Strega 2015). I became a committed social justice worker; I did not want the research to follow a standard social science model. I wanted the voice as part of the ongoing conversation not marginalised to its own chapter, tied down and then silenced. Armed with advice from Potts and Brown (2015, p. 37):

> You will encounter these discourses, and it will be up to you to understand the deep positivist and neoliberal epistemological roots they extend from. You will need to see how these discourses will try to construct and constrain your work. And, most importantly, you will need to know how to engage anti-oppressive practices to try and produce social justice outcomes despite the constraints.

The work of Brown and Strega (2005, 2015) was supportive of my ideas and encouraged me to stand up for different ways of knowing and story-telling. I am a story-teller, and I needed to tell the IMG story from the voices I had been gifted. Brown and Strega (2005, p. 2) see research as resistance and the intention is:

> To make space and take space for marginalized researchers and ideas. We push the edges of academic acceptability not because we want to be accepted within the academy but in order to transform it.

In fact, Strega (2015, p. 144), referring especially to academic institutions points out that: "Historical and critical analysis of the role of research in marginalized lives makes us aware that these institutions are also deeply implicated in maintaining and rationalizing inequities". Through the processes of field work, the data collection and the emerging media content, analysis with social justice at its heart, were fuelled by constant questioning, reflexivity and comprehensively revisiting the data.

Power emerged as the first major player, firstly the power invested in and exercised through the health system with the medical profession as gatekeepers. Secondly, the concept of medical dominance and how it works to maintain the power of the medical profession, thoroughly theorised by Willis (1989, 2006) was illuminating and assisted with conceptualising structures and power relationships. To gain further understanding, an historical lens was required to aid in understanding the present following Mills (1959) the study required history and biography.

## The First IMGs

The first IMGs in Australia were introduced as British naval surgeons, nine of whom arrived via the first fleet in 1788, and doctor explorers who accompanied expeditions to map the Australian coast. What these adventurers came to was an ancient land populated with many Indigenous nations and language groups (Foley 2008). The invaders had no idea of the complex social systems they were displacing and quickly dismissed the black people they saw as heathens and savages (Hirst 2014). Post-British invasion, this ancient land began to take a different shape with the marginalisation of the traditional peoples, massacres and progressive dispossession from their land (Breen 2008). Through the process of colonisation, Indigenous Australians became regarded as and subsequently oppressed by a race category. They were classified within that category on the basis of full bloods or various levels of mixed blood (Hirst 2014; Kidd 2008). Although Australia's new population was a motley crew of convicts and military personnel, white supremacy reigned. 1788 marked the beginning of the Australia we know today, a xenophobic, ethnocentric and racist country. Evidence of this can be found in the current government's: Operation Sovereign Borders initiative (Department of Immigration and Border Protection 2016). Australians are fearful and suspicious of the other, tend to believe that our way of life, norms and values is superior to those of others and prefer to keep Indigenous Australians and other undesirable races as invisible as possible because we want to be a country populated by white, English-speaking citizens who have British ancestry. There are a number of blights on Australia's 'goodness' over time such as the White Australia Policy which was trumpeted in conjunction with the establishment of the great nation state Australia at Federation in 1901 (Gunstone 2017). This blatantly racist policy institutionalised racism and made it very clear to the world that the vision for the new nation was a white one. Australia's non-acceptance of overseas medical qualifications first arose when doctors arrived from Europe as displaced persons after the Second World War (Iredale 2009; Kunz 1975). There is an interesting connection here in that Australia's population at the time needed boosting and immigration was being championed as a means to do this. This initiative arose out of a xenophobic fear that Australia, with a small population, could be invaded from the North by hordes of Asians (Hirst 2014). The connection here is echoed in Australia today, in that we need to boost the medical workforce, particularly in rural and remote areas, by actively recruiting health professionals from overseas. When they come, however, the standard of their qualifications is assumed deficient. They are subjected to overzealous assessment or banished to the medical unemployed. Grigg and Manderson (2016, p. 13) in their paper tracing the development of the Australian Racism, Acceptance and Cultural-Ethnocentrism scale (RACES) confirm that:

> Racism is a significant challenge in contemporary Australian society due to the potential and significant negative impact on a range of health, social, psychological, and economic outcomes of the diverse racial, ethnic, cultural, and religious groups within Australia.

Similarly, the National Mental Health Survey of Doctors and Medical Students conducted by Beyond Blue (2013) found that IMGs identified and reported racism as a source of work-related stress. In addition, Knowles (2015, p. 4) found that twenty-seven percent of IMGs reported racial discrimination. In their submission to the 2016 Senate Community Affairs References Committee Inquiry, the Australian Indigenous Doctors' Association (AIDA) (2016, submission 8) reported that Indigenous Australian medical doctors experience racial discrimination during their training and subsequent practice. This manifested in racist behaviours from colleagues and "systemic racism embedded in the institutions they work in and under" (AIDA 2016, submission 8, p. 2).

The white Australia policy was abolished in the 1960s by the Whitlam Labour Government (Hirst 2014) and gave way to multiculturalism. Abolishing or, for that matter, introducing policy does not ensure that the minds and behaviours of the general public and institutions are instantaneously reformed, and this is evidenced above. Moreover, multiculturalism sent a message that Australians embrace cultural diversity. Multiculturalism was a project to reimagine a national identity, one that would accommodate migrants from different backgrounds. Australians, however, perhaps just tolerated multiculturalism, rather than genuinely accepted it (Plage et al. 2016). An historical perspective explored, it was necessary to turn focus back to the power structures of today with the knowledge of some of the contributing factors to their creation. The structure and play of power in IMG relations with the health system and the Australian medical profession were unpacked, essentially, a macro-analysis of the system and micro-analysis of the individual narratives of IMG experiences.

## Power Dimensions

Foucault's extensive work on power and knowledge was helpful here to provide clarity to what was unfolding. Foucault (1997) believed that by understanding how power works as an instrument of discourse, we can in turn uncover how human life is situated within discourse and then how, as a result, discourse rules and governs humans (Wang 2017). The power differential and power struggles at the sight of the power/knowledge nexus became a major focus as IMG narratives revealed their experiences. Power struggles establish the meaning in discourse and the resulting effect of power that which becomes regarded as truth. In her discussion of Foucault's work, Macias (2015, pp. 238–239) emphasises the: "Need to pay attention to the conditions that make truth a product of discourse and power. The power struggles to grant some statements more validity than others". The positioning of IMGs as an underclass within the elite profession of medicine is embedded in a deficit discourse which communicates to IMGs a perceived inferiority of their qualifications and skills.

Following Hill Collins (2000), relations were presented in terms of a matrix of domination. Relations of power and associated discourses are structured into structural, hegemonic and interpersonal power domains to enable insight into how IMGs are positioned within Australia's medical culture. Structural power is represented by the system and its many agencies as well as the numerous processes IMGs are required to negotiate. From obtaining the most suitable visa, gaining accreditation and registration to finding employment, all processes involve IMG/system interaction. The confusing array of pathway choices for IMGs has been outlined, as well as the racist initiative of the competent authority pathway, an option available only to IMGs from selected countries. Hegemonic power refers to the Australian medical profession specifically and its power, influence and control as gatekeepers to the health system. The third dimension of power is interpersonal power. This power category is concerned with the voices of IMGs and their relationships and discourses with the system and with the Australian medical profession. The reality of lived experience for IMGs in Australia is controlled by numerous identities which take the form of agencies, professional bodies, government departments and the like. The medical colleges, of which there are sixteen, regulate entry into the specialties. Medicare issues provider numbers while visas are the responsibility of the Department of Immigration and Border Protection (Harris 2009). Through this complex bureaucracy of structural power, IMGs are classified, regulated, managed and controlled as the other; medical doctors trained overseas. The hegemonic positioning of the medical profession as gatekeepers to the structural power of the system cements together a mutually beneficial power alliance. Hegemonic power allows the medical profession to maintain a self-interest agenda which drives the need to "other" IMGs, rather than the espoused rhetoric of the need to maintain high standards. The structural power/hegemonic power alliance is a long-standing relationship which by 1880 saw medicine developing an elite status (Willis 1989, p. 60).

The interpersonal power dimension in the matrix of domination draws the voice into the conversation, and what is revealed is predominantly a power struggle, interpersonal power relations with the structural power of the system and the hegemonic power of the medical profession. IMGs share their rich narratives of lived experience and the reader is able to gain an appreciation of the gamut of emotions and experiences revealed. Among them, there is distress and frustration, career aspirations ruined and an adverse impact on mental and physical health. In fact, the mental health of doctors generally has been a concern for some time. A key finding of the 2013 survey into the mental health of medical doctors in Australia revealed that: "Doctors reported substantially higher rates of psychological distress and attempted suicide compared to both the Australian population and other Australian professions" (Beyond Blue 2013, p. 2). IMGs carry additional stress due to the extra demands that the system requires of them, because they are not Australian trained.

Various strategies of control and vehicles for exclusion are mentioned such as examinations and fees. Failure at exams denies IMG's access to progression through the required processes; in addition if an IMG is not financially able, he or she may not be able to sit exams at all. Progression through the system attracts a myriad of fees; an IMG must be able to finance these. If an IMG is unemployed without reasonable savings, he or she is not only significantly disadvantaged but excluded. The considerable hegemonic power held by the Australian medical profession is extended and developed into the concept of medical dominance.

## Medical Dominance and Toxic Tales

The concept of medical dominance equates to a control of esoteric knowledge which is maintained by the interface between the economy and the State. Interested in the division of labour in the health system, the work of Willis (1989) mapped the parameters of medical dominance to extend to: dominance over the practice of medicine, over the work of other healthcare providers and over society. Medical dominance enables the exclusion of complementary and alternate health therapies. Despite the growing popularity of these therapies, medical dominance ensures that they remain marginalised (Twohig 2016). The rise of the profession of medicine from the 1870s when medicine attained scientific status is explored to put context around the development of medical dominance, and how it has changed over time.

Currently, medical dominance is being challenged from various quarters and is changing shape to accommodate itself within changing healthcare delivery practice (Coburn 2006; Germov 2014; Willis 2006). For example, since the 1990s a more corporate style of control of health service delivery has developed in general practice. There is an increased focus on managerialism, regulation of work practices and accountability. A major change agent has been the growth of digital health technologies and there have been changes in the doctor/patient relationship (Duckett 2008; Willis et al. 2016). For example, the Internet has transformed access to general medical advice and information for patients, while doctors now expect patients to take more responsibility for their own health. Ultimately, despite challenges and the need to give concessions here and there, medical dominance is still alive and well. The medical profession, however, is sometimes at odds with the State. Germov (2014, p. 399) views the current changes as a battle with the State:

> Clinical governance heralds an era where the performance of individual doctors and hospitals can potentially be publicly comparable in terms of cost, timeliness, and clinical standards of effective treatment outcomes. It is an attempt by the state to exercise control over the medical profession at the clinical level-the last bastion of medical dominance.

Currently in Australia, there are three major power players in health: the government which holds the authority, medicine which has the professional knowledge and clinical skills and the private sector (Willis et al. 2016). Medicine's power therefore remains immense, simply because it holds the status of institutionalised expert, the keeper of knowledge that the other players do not have. Against this backdrop, however, the reader has the opportunity to learn about the ugly side of medicine, the institutionalised expert with a great deal of power, status and respect has been tarnished and the reputation of medicine is called into question. During 2015, numerous adverse reports around medicine's endemic, unsavoury culture surfaced in the Australian media. Some of the voices from the stories shared with the media were invited to join the IMGs voices already shared from the data set of this study (the focus group, individual interviews, the 2012 Parliamentary Inquiry and the 2016 Senate Community Affairs References Committee) because they are also voices in crisis, from within a profession in crisis. The voices from the media too had some shocking and disturbing stories to share. These included a plea from the then Australian Medical Students' Association president, James Lawler (Campus Review 2015) following four medical student suicides in the first half of 2015. Lawler appealed to senior medical practitioners to step up and stop bullying behaviours. In its investigation into the mental health of doctors, Beyond Blue (2013, p. 5) established that: "Medical students reported high rates of general and specific distress in comparison to the general population". In addition to bullying, the ABC's *4 Corners* program presented by Kerry O'Brien on the 25th May 2015 reported claims that belittling and bastardisation were: "poisoning the lives of young trainee doctors in teaching hospitals" (McDermott 2015). Reports of sexism and sexual harassment were rife, particularly in the surgical fields and again particularly within hospitals. A young female trainee surgeon commented that because she had refused the sexual advances of her supervisor her career was now over. It was also mentioned that to report incidents ultimately resulted in career suicide (Knowles 2015). Another mentioned that in the workplace, she suffered humiliation every day. There are many examples of sexism directed towards women within medicine. Often these examples involved women being relegated to the domestic stereotypes associated with the kitchen/grocery domain or to the sexual body image/fertility domain. For example, two specific episodes of blatant sexism and harassment were offered to the RACS expert panel by female trainee surgeons. The first was a demeaning comment made by a male senior surgeon to a female trainee who thought she was going to be invited to assist him in surgery: "Why don't you just go and do the grocery shopping…or you can join us in theatre—not to do anything, just for eye candy". Another female trainee surgeon seeking a job stated: "I was told I would only be considered for the job if I had my tubes tied" (Knowles 2015, p. 12). The Royal Australasian College of Surgeons appointed expert advisory panel's subsequent report found that in terms of discrimination, bullying and sexual harassment: "It is inconceivable that anyone finds this acceptable or contests the seriousness and spread of these problems" (2015, p. 3). It is not surprising then that a profession with an established toxic culture has no qualms in positioning IMGs as an underclass and also subjecting them to aspects of toxicity.

These startling findings beg the question of possible retaliation. As discriminatory, bullying and sexual harassment behaviours are against the law; it could be only a matter of time before legal action such as a class action is instigated against the RACS, other medical speciality colleges or individual medical practitioners. Has the medical profession/Australian community relationship been damaged? I argue it has. While the medical profession may possess considerable power and status it has also shown the weakness within, the outcome of a weak professional culture one of bullying, sexual harassment and self-interest is, instead, power failure.

IMGs are often viewed as some kind of a problem or at least problematic, yet they have come to Australia to assist with a problem, that of a health workforce shortage. Analysis suggests why IMGs are positioned as an underclass within an elite profession. This requires closer questioning of problem representations and the teasing out of any associated silences. Initially, a global representation of IMGs is investigated as in today's world there is a climate of vast international exchange between nations, from ideas and technologies to goods and services. As a result, there is an international migration of the workforce (Toader and Sfetcu 2013). The medical profession is no exception and the supply of medical doctors varies around the world.

# Migration as an Ethical Dilemma

Medical doctors are a valuable resource, highly sought after by countries experiencing a health workforce shortage (such as Australia). Countries in need of more medical doctors actively recruit them from elsewhere. However, there is concern associated with wealthy, developed countries 'poaching' doctors from poor, underdeveloped countries (OECD 2015). This practice is not confined to poor source countries supplying wealthier host countries, however, and developed countries also lure doctors from other developed countries. There are two dilemmas here: firstly, the freedom of doctors and, secondly, the idea of compensation. The free movement of human beings is considered a basic human right, and therefore regardless of where they have trained, medical doctors are human beings and should be free to migrate to any country of their choice anywhere in the world. This leaves the source country without those medical doctors. The question then becomes: should the host country somehow compensate the source country? Some developed countries have undertaken to cease recruitment of IMGs from underdeveloped countries. The issue of compensation is a difficult one to establish and would possibly need a country by country approach. It has been noted (Dwyer 2007; Iredale 2009; Smith 2008) that host countries are reluctant to undertake compensation discussions. Why do IMGs decide to migrate?

# Risk-Taking for Safety

The voices join the conversation and explain their reasons for coming to Australia. They share their need to feel safe for themselves and their families as well as the perceived opportunities offered in Australia. Linked to these desires is discussion around safety and psychological stress, with some IMGs arriving in Australia already psychologically vulnerable due to their traumatic experiences of war, political uncertainty and persecution (Kahn et al. 2015). Human rights and refugees are also explored and the problematic representation of IMGs. The wicked problem concept (a problem which is highly resistant to a solution) and problem representation present a framework for useful exploration and clarification by employing Bacchi's (2009): "What's the problem represented to be approach". Following Bacchi's (2009) six question model systematically, it is argued that there is no real problem with IMGs, rather the problems lie with the injustices and inefficiencies in the system's dealings with IMGs. The silences have been in medicine's toxic culture, now thoroughly exposed. Bacchi (2009) advocates a paradigm shift from a problem-solving focus to a problem-questioning approach. This allows space for consideration of the problem fallout, the possible impact on those involved, how they are treated and how they feel about themselves. IMGs are met with a deficit discourse from the moment they attempt to come to Australia, immediately they are in a position of constantly having to prove themselves, the standard of their qualifications and the competency of their clinical skills. At the same time, many who have difficulties with accreditation and registration are faced with the challenge of retaining their dignity, self-esteem and medical identity.

I argue that the analytic tool of intersectionality represents an effective multidisciplinary vehicle for critical inquiry and praxis, as the approach seeks to confront unjust power relations (Hill Collins and Bilge 2016; Hill Collins and Solomos 2010). Particularly suited for analysis in this research study, intersectionality is fluid in that the intersecting oppressions of class, race and nation are not fixed, rather they weave their way within and through each other. In order to empower IMGs with a sense of solidarity and shared purpose (Sefa Dei 2008), they are represented as a community construct that is a professional community that shares an occupation (Hill Collins 2010). I did not want to disempower the IMG community by separating out divisions from within such as gender and ethnicity (while many intersectionality studies use these categories and they are very important). IMGs have enough to contend with in Australia; therefore, I sought to facilitate solidarity in IMG agency. The system with which the IMG community must engage represents a manifestation of Australian 'normalcy'. Entrenched within the system and operationalised via its discourses and structures is structural violence and systemic bias (Galtung 1990) coupled with a systemic frustration of aspirations (Eckermann et al. 2006). The current political climate begins discussion around the intersecting inequalities of class, race and nation and their influence on the positioning of IMGs. The political climate provides a feel for how Australian citizens are voting, and as a result, how governments are reflecting the will of the people by passing legislation of ideas, policies and processes into laws, and subsequently into institutional structures. These laws and institutions are the sites of struggle for IMGs and provide a picture of the Australian nation and what it stands for. Recently, however, there is a shift to a political right-wing conservative stance which is represented in Australia, the USA, the UK and emerging in Europe. There are common threads which link the shifts that have been brought about by an angry voter backlash. There is also a commonality of the element of surprise in these results. Concerns around the economy, immigration and jobs, the maintenance of national identity and a nostalgic return to 'greatness' are all central to this political movement. This sentiment is indicative to a common reluctance to embrace the transformations associated with modern life, as outlined by Blackshaw (2010, p. 146):

> The two concepts of nostalgia and community are indelibly connected as they simultaneously evoke the idea of a past that is committed to memory on the basis of both enchantment and appetite…in this coming together of community and nostalgia, there is a strong connection between the themes of loss, longing, regret and suffering.

The vote in the UK to leave the European Union (Brexit) shocked many. A champion of the leave vote, Nigel Farage, expressed nostalgic great nation sentiment (Chang 2016). Farage has openly been accused of racist and xenophobic views (Armstrong and Britton 2016) and publicly backed Australia's tough immigration policy (Chang 2016). Similarly, the election of Donald Trump to the presidency of the USA stunned many around the world. Trump has promised to fix an ailing US economy by 'making America great again'. For Trump, tight restrictions, or in some cases bans on immigration (particularly Muslims) will help bring back jobs and safety for Americans. In Australia, Pauline Hanson's One Nation Party has re-emerged as a viable option for voters and was even preferred by the Liberal Party in a recent West Australian election. Hanson expressed her delight at the Brexit vote and Trump's election via twitter. Hanson, a nationalist advocate, has been outspoken over several years expressing racist, xenophobic and ethnocentric views. She has demonised Australia's Indigenous peoples, Asians and now Muslims. Hanson has warned that unless Australia stops Muslim immigration and bans the burqa, Australians will find themselves living under Sharia law (One Nation Party 2016). This political climate is likely to spread and it is an uncomfortable time for immigration, including IMGs currently in Australia, and those who desire to come to Australia. The right-wing political phenomenon is not new and emerges as the result of constant class struggle. The Precariat class advanced by Standing (2011) offers a possible profile for those who become disenfranchised in society. The Precariat is a frustrated and angry group without agency or security. Their precarious position, due to increasing casualization of the workforce and decline in full-time jobs and careers, has become normalised in globalised labour markets. Many IMGs find themselves in similar circumstances while they await the system's decision on accreditation and registration. Some join the ranks of the medical unemployed, driving taxis and delivering pizza. IMGs receive mixed messages; Australia can be espoused as a free egalitarian society, where there is a 'fair go' for all (Plage et al. 2016). Simultaneously, Australia in reality offers only a 'fair go' for some. Demonstrated throughout this book is Australia's long history of racism, xenophobia and ethnocentricism. Currently, around the world there is an immigration crisis, the like of which has not been seen since Second World War, and as a result, there are growing tensions. People are fleeing from war, poverty and persecution especially from the Middle East and Africa. Many of these people are seeking asylum from countries without the infrastructure to accommodate refugees, and many of these people have no choice but to embark on perilous sea voyages (Brannan et al. 2016). Tragically, there have been many drownings. I argue that Australia has developed paranoia around people fleeing to Australia via boat and has gone to great lengths to ensure that these people do not set foot on Australian soil. Australian Detention Centres located elsewhere have become the 'new home' for refugees and asylum seekers while they await acceptance and resettlement (Maley 2016). These locations have been described as constituting concentration camps. The rhetoric around stopping people smugglers bringing desperate people in often unsafe boats is presented as humanitarian concern due to lives lost at sea, but the conditions provided for these people in the detention centres are not humane. In its most extreme display of xenophobic policy yet, the Australian government has determined that detainees on the Islands at any time since the second half of 2013 will never be accepted in Australia under any circumstances (not even as a tourist) for the rest of their lives (Riley 2016). There is a fear that once a detainee is resettled in another country he or she may again attempt to come to Australia. Australia seems determined to evade the humanitarian crisis on its door step and sends a message to the world that asylum seekers and refugees are not welcome. In their discussion on neoliberalism and nationalism in Australia, Lueck et al. (2015, p. 612) note that:

> Assylum seekers are frequently politicized in media discourses, that is, presented within the framework of politics rather than for instance, human rights, and that this includes little self-representation or humanization.

Racism is often a partner of xenophobia, and from 1788, racism has been manifested in Australian society based on an ethnocentric perception of racial superiority. The British invasion of 1788 resulted in the decimation of the first peoples' knowledge, cultures and traditions which were deemed inferior. This began Australia's poor human rights record. The participation of Indigenous Australians in Australian society is still steeped in a Western discourse which positions the first peoples within a 'race' social construct (Foley 2008). Colour and racial/ethnic origins can be assigned to both white and black people. However, the outcome is very different; for blacks, there are disadvantages, but for whites the outcome is privilege (Moreton-Robinson 2004). Some IMGs have shared their perceptions of the black/white binary, and the outcome for IMGs with black skin is perhaps a double or extra burden of difference. From the very beginnings of the 'new' nation, Australia has strived for a white nation. Discussion highlights whiteness as power and privilege, and whiteness is the normative epistemology. A blatant, ongoing example of institutionalised racism in Australia is Indigenous Australian disadvantage and the chronic policy failure to address it. This has, in itself, become a wicked problem with no solution in sight. IMGs and Indigenous Australian medical doctors experience racism in daily life and in workplaces and was identified to the 2016 Senate Community Affairs References Committee on Medical Complaints process in Australia as a source of workplace stress. Racism is institutionalised and anti-immigration sentiment comes directly from the government. In fact, at the time of writing (2017), the prime minister has proposed changes to section 18C of the Racial Discrimination Act. At a joint party room meeting, the race-hate laws will be watered down in the interests of freedom of speech. "Offend, insult and humiliate" will be replaced by "harass and intimidate" making racial discrimination claims harder to prove. The Shadow Attorney General, Dreyfus (2017) commented in a press conference that: "Every single ethnic community in Australia has been betrayed by this government". Currently, Indigenous Australians are not included in the Australian constitution and the government is stalling on the idea of a referendum for our inclusion. There is a tension between the rejection of Indigenous sovereignty by Australian governments and Indigenous Australians claim that sovereignty has never been surrendered (Gunstone 2007). A no vote in a referendum to include Indigenous Australians in the constitution would be disastrous for Australia.

What do IMGs make of these mixed messages? Australia is experiencing a health workforce shortage and IMGs are encouraged to bring their experience and skills to Australia, but what kind of country is Australia? The Australian nation appears to be at odds with itself; on the one hand, there is the image of a 'fair go for all', an egalitarian land of milk and honey. On the other hand, there is the image of a nation which excludes Indigenous Australians and tolerates the fact that many

Indigenous Australians live in Third-World conditions and experience the poorest health of any group in the country. However, the majority of the Australian population enjoy a First-World health system (Reid et al. 2016). In addition, Australia's anti-immigration stance is the toughest in the world and sends a clear message that people fleeing dire circumstances are not welcome (Riley 2016). Moreover, IMGs who come to Australia must deal with a dysfunctional system and endure the toxic culture of the medical profession. Australia is clearly not the country it imagines itself to be. Despite numerous inquiries which acknowledge the shortcomings of the system and its processes, the difficulties faced by many IMGs persist.

## Let us Have Another Inquiry

The evidence that generally a wicked problem exists within the system and medicine's culture, is confirmed by the string of inquiries. For decades, all manner of inquiries related to IMGs, medical workforce supply, assessment processes and complaints associated with medicine and the like have been undertaken. No real solutions have come out of these. Issues are exposed; subsequent recommendations are made but very little if anything really changes. Susskind and Susskind (2015, p. 37) clarify the context:

> When confronted with the criticisms and challenges…a common response of professionals (and their representative bodies) is to address each alleged shortcoming in turn and to suggest small modifications. The mindset here is to repair the traditional way of working.

An examination of these inquiries reveals a repetitive discourse around recommendations, with terms such as accountability, transparency and efficiency strongly featured. There are possible new inquiries on the horizon too, as suggested in recommendation six of the 2016 Senate Community Affairs References Committee Inquiry. The committee suggests a further inquiry into the medical complaints process and the National Law. What will become of another inquiry remains to be seen, what does remain however, is the ongoing difficulties experienced by IMGs in their dealings with the system and the toxic culture within Australian medicine. I argue that the powerful medical profession has succumbed to the weakness within, and as a result, there is power failure. The profession is in breach of its service to the community. Therefore, I argue that the toxic culture of medicine and the associated totally unacceptable behaviours render the social contract broken; medicine is in breach of contract.

## A Breach of Social Contract

After a toxic culture is unearthed, how is it addressed? Can it be managed and eliminated? Does a toxic culture represent a wicked problem, one that is highly resistant to a solution? When the voices of those who have suffered at the hands of some misguided individuals within the profession, or at the hands of the health system, or at the hands of various associated bodies speak, it is a powerful voice. It is difficult to marry the 'social contract' proposed by Susskind and Susskind (2015) (also see Sen 2010) to the behaviours exhibited by sectors of the medical profession. It seems that the profession does not fulfil all the obligations associated with their suggested end of the bargain.

The Australian public did not agree in good faith for medical professionals to look after their own interests first and foremost, nor did they agree for the esteemed profession to produce bullying, sexual harassment and unlawful practices which in some cases, have led to victims taking their lives. The Australian public deserve better as do those who have suffered and continue to suffer. The medical students trained in a bullying culture, through "pedagogy of humiliation" (AMSA 2016 Submission 10, p. 6) did not enter university with the intent to become the next generation of bullies. The IMGs, who have been denied the opportunity to utilise their skills and those who have been forced to compromise those skills in order to gain some employment, are innocent victims. Where are these IMGs and how do they retain their agency and medical identity as fully qualified medical doctors? The study by Harris and Guillemin (2015, p. 169) established that IMGs working to obtain registration constitute a medical underground and enterprisingly utilise peripheral spaces within a hospital to maintain and strengthen identity:

> One group of IMGs gathered regularly in this cafeteria on Sundays to study for the written exam, amidst containers of homemade cake and photocopied papers. Dr Rudi van Aarde, a clinically retired IMG who had worked for 30 years as a general practitioner in Johannesburg and still attended the Sunday session, spoke about the members of this group. He talked about the leader of the group who had worked in Kuwait, Egypt, London, Ireland, Scandinavia and New Zealand before coming to Australia. He talked about the German psychiatrist, the Indian oncologist and an Eritrean general practitioner, a paediatric surgeon who was working as a hospital cleaner, another working as a nurse. He said that there was an Afghani cardiologist there too and a doctor working as a night watchman. Many IMGs in this group were a lot older than those on the wards; they were rich with years of previous clinical experience. The Sunday group was struggling to pass a written medical exam modelled on that given to final year medical students in Australia. Many of these IMGs were in a holding pattern, waiting and hoping to find a place in the Australian medical profession.

These IMGs struggle to retain a community solidarity which affirms their identity as medical practitioners. Some may succeed and become registered medical practitioners in Australia with employment in their chosen speciality and some may not. What will medicine itself become in a changing future?

## What of the Future?

Susskind and Susskind (2015) have predicted that technological advances will transform the professions, including medicine well into the future. They do explain however that there will be resistance such as old entrenched ideas will be hard to abandon, an attachment to the way we always do things and perhaps a stubbornness to accept that another way could be better. The medical profession could well suffer from what they call 'technological myopia':

> A tendency to underestimate the potential of tomorrow's applications by evaluating them in terms of today's enabling technologies....this is the inability of a sceptic, because of the shortcoming of current technology, to concede that future systems may be radically more powerful than those of today. (Susskind and Susskind 2015, p. 44)

Is this in fact the road to a kind of technological determinism, a world of unfeeling machines, robots, devices? Where is the human? Important conversations need to take place around not only the advantages of technological determinism but also the disadvantages. In terms of medical care for example, who could be marginalised or even excluded? Individually, perhaps the poor, the elderly, those with impairments would be disadvantaged. In terms of communities, perhaps rural or remote communities and Indigenous communities would be disadvantaged. Some of these communities may have no, limited or unreliable Internet access.

However, perhaps Artificial Intelligence (AI) holds the key to a marriage between humanness and technology. The academic community has expressed warning about the potential dangers of AI, but also highlights the potential benefits. Speaking at the opening of the Leverhulme Centre for the Future of Intelligence (LCFI) at Cambridge University, the late Professor Stephen Hawking (2016) noted that AI could be the best or worst thing to happen to humanity:

> Perhaps with the tools of this new technological revolution, we will be able to undo some of the damage done to the natural world by the last one – industrialisation. And surely we will aim to finally eradicate disease and poverty. (Hern 2016)

A world without disease and poverty would certainly be a challenge to the medical profession. Could technological change push medical dominance to the point where it no longer exists? Or conversely, could medical dominance become even more powerful, further empowered with the assistance of new technologies? Could the position of IMGs become empowered by technological change and take on another status? However, Friedson (1994) reminds that while there is even greater, continuing change ahead, self-interest is a human trait and will remain. The negatives of medical dominance will only be eliminated if it is liberated from material self-interest. Given the existing circumstances, this seems highly unlikely for this powerful profession. In fact, Baudrillard (2010, p. 17) suggests that power has to be eliminated altogether, where both sovereign and subject reject domination: "It is power itself that has to be abolished—and not just in refusal *to be dominated*, which is the essence of all traditional struggles, but equally and as violently in the refusal to *dominate*". The power differential within medicine in Australia, however, appears fixed at this time. The work of Nobel Prize winner Amartya Sen around social justice and reason places the role of institutions as instrumental in the pursuit of justice. He argues that institutional involvement allows for the possibility of several different reasonable stances or positions. However, what is certain is that: "at a particular time not everyone is willing to undertake such scrutiny". Reasoned justice is often avoided by: "placid guardians of order and justice" (Sen 2010, p. 7). For Sullivan (2016, p. 1) "Social

justice demands equity in health capability more than equal access to health services".
Ultimately, it is fundamental for the population to feel empowered to manage its
health and have confidence in health services and in the professionals who work
in them. Perhaps an optimal/maximal approach has potential? According to Sen
(2016, p. 1): "Critical sound reasoning can lead us to a partial ordering yielding a
maximal alternative that is not optimal". The voices gifted to this study have spoken
out about their experiences and observations. From these narratives, it seems that
the medical profession and the toxic culture within is underpinned and influenced by
several negative factors: the profession is hierarchically structured and entrenched
with gender and cultural stereotypes.

There is a power imbalance and competitive nature embedded in medical training
and medical practice. As a result, there is an environment conducive to negative
behaviours. Surely, the moral and the material are inextricably linked:

> And, as such, [we] must recognise love as an essential ingredient of a just society…love is a
> political principle through which we struggle to create mutually life-enhancing opportunities
> for all people. It is grounded in the mutuality and interdependence of our human existence-
> that which we share, as much as that which we do not. This is a love nurtured by the act
> of relationship itself. It cultivates relationships with the freedom to be at one's best without
> undue fear. Such an emancipatory love allows us to realize our nature in a way that allows
> others to do so as well. Inherent in such a love is the understanding that we are not at liberty
> to be violent, authoritarian, or self-seeking. (Darder and Miron 2006; Denzin and Lincoln
> 2008, p. 152)

I have been left disturbed by the toxic culture within medicine itself and by what
is happening in the nation of Australia. This nation recruits IMGs to serve our health
workforce needs and then treats them shabbily. In our interview, Barry expressed his
opinion by touching on what he saw as the fundamental, underpinning problem:

Barry explained succinctly his perception of what underpins the situation as a
whole:

> They know they need us to help out, there aren't enough doctors here. But they wish they
> didn't need us, that is the problem. They don't want us here so they try to make it as hard as
> they can for us. The government says we should come but they [Australian trained doctors]
> want to keep us out. (2011, interview 6)

Australia has a border protection agenda that is xenophobic in the extreme and
Indigenous Australians are subjected to institutionalised racism (Gunstone 2017).
The intersecting inequalities of class, race and nation in Australia conspire to relegate IMGs to an underclass within the Australian medical profession. The contribution to the literature made here clearly demonstrates the positioning of IMGs. Why
IMGs are positioned as such is advanced, adding to the existing literature around
medical dominance. The groundbreaking work of Willis (1989) began the research
to explain how medical dominance is established and maintained, much scholarship
has followed (Coburn 2006; Coburn and Willis 2000; Germov 2014; Keleher 2016;
Willis 2006) and within that scholarship medical dominance has been found to be
accommodating change while retaining its position. The gap in the literature which
this book has now consolidated is twofold. Firstly, the positioning of IMGs specifically within medical dominance as a discrete community of medical practitioners

ascribed a lower-class status. Secondly, the question of why IMGs have come to be positioned as an underclass within an elite profession has been explored. I believe the current circumstances surrounding IMGs and Australia's medical culture constitute a wicked problem. Significant, robust change in attitudes and values on the part of resistant individuals and organisations is a difficult and complex project, and further, how major change could be successfully brought about is also complex. What is clear however, is that medicine in Australia is imploding due to a power failure brought about by itself. However, just because the current culture within medicine seems insurmountable does not mean that no attempt should be made to begin to address it.

Something must be done. There is too much at stake to allow the continuation of a toxic culture which potentially threatens patient safety, IMGs, medical students and medical doctors of all specialities. In their discussion of wicked problems from a national perspective, Newman and Head (2017, p. 40) point out that: "the very fact that the concept of wicked problems has caught the attention of public policy scholars signifies that there is some belief that potential remedies exist". There are many medical professionals who do not condone or practice toxic behaviours. The Royal Australasian College of Surgeons is leading the way towards change, currently working on recommendations made by the Expert Advisory Group on discrimination, bullying and sexual harassment (Knowles 2015). The Advisory Group conducted research across Australia and New Zealand and found that: "The problems exist across all surgical specialities in both countries and in all regions and senior surgeons and surgical consultants are reported as the primary source of these problems" (Knowles 2015, p. 4).

Further, in their statement to the college, the Advisory Group acknowledged that: "It will take a collective recognition that there must be a profound shift in the culture of surgery and an unwavering commitment to achieving this" (p. 2). Ultimately, the Group asserted that:

- Every patient has a right to expect that their health care is uncompromised by discrimination, bullying and sexual harassment in surgery.
- Every surgical trainee has a right to an education free of discrimination, bullying and sexual harassment.
- Every IMG has a right to be assessed on their merits, free of discrimination, bullying and sexual harassment (p. 2).

Surgery is certainly not the only medical field where these problems exist, in fact the health sector as a whole has been identified, but surgery, in particular, has been singled out as harbouring the worst for these behaviours which have become long-standing and therefore normalised. Knowles (2015, p. 2) confirms:

Long established traditions that have been inherited and have normalised unprofessional, and sometimes illegal, behaviours must be relinquished. Gender inequity must be addressed. Discrimination, bullying and sexual harassment must become problems of the past.

Given this situation, it seems useful to begin with medical education, as it is here where the teaching of the culture begins. If medical students must witness and tolerate unacceptable behaviours, effectively the next generation for the perpetuation of these behaviours is being groomed. Graduating students will then become the next generation to teach and carry out these behaviours. This is incongruent with what is officially desired and purported to be the case by universities, hence confirming that robust action is required. For example, the president of Medical Deans Australia and New Zealand, Professor Murray (2017) stated:

> Medical Deans are on record in asserting that all medical students deserve to study medicine free from bullying, fear and discrimination. Universities and medical schools have clear policies on these matters.

Medical Deans Australia and New Zealand have established a working group committed to medical student health and well-being. By graduation, medical students are expected to have achieved outstanding professional values. For example, the AMC graduate outcome statement 4.2 (Medical Deans Australia and New Zealand 2017, p.15) requires the medical graduate to:

> Demonstrate professional values including commitment to high quality clinical standards, compassion, empathy and respect for all patients. Demonstrate the qualities of integrity, honesty, leadership and partnership to patients, the profession and society.

Clearly, there is a problem here and there is much work to do to ensure policy transfers into action. Universities and medical schools need to be held to account for their duty of care responsibilities to students. Similarly, hospitals must also be held to account to provide safe workplaces for all who work and train there. If real, genuine transformation is desired, and then it must come from all quarters and have the support of all stakeholders. Any changes must have powerful institutionalised back up within government policies and legislation. According to Knowles (2015, p. 3), a monumental shift across the board will be required to deconstruct the existing context:

> There is no room for bystanders. Employers, hospitals, governments, health professional and Industrial associations, regulators and other partners in the health sector must also commit to sustained action. It will take employers taking seriously their responsibilities to provide a safe workplace and governments supporting hospitals to do this. It will take new partnerships, committed collaboration and fresh approaches.

Graduate outcomes must also be championed off paper and into reality. The culture of a medical school must model, teach, develop and nurture the qualities to enable students to achieve them. Medical educators and those who provide supervision to trainees and IMGs should be required to undertake training in the field of Adult Learning to raise awareness of equitable and respectful training strategies. Ideally, this training would facilitate and support those involved to become more effective teachers. In addition, training in cultural competence/safety would equip medical educators and supervisors to become more aware and empathic of IMGs and Indigenous Australians, their backgrounds and needs. The training and assessment of IMGs should be independently and externally scrutinised to avoid discrimination. Medical Deans must be empowered to act on code of conduct violations, and hospitals and universities need to be empowered to enforce disciplinary action against perpetrators. Violations should be linked to and embedded in performance review and penalties apply for inappropriate behaviours.

There is also a culture of fear of reprisal around making complaints and reporting inappropriate behaviours, or even mentioning concerns. The problem is evidenced throughout this book. A safe and confidential space and process needs to be created where all complainants: "Can complain even against the person at the top and not have to worry about losing their career" (Knowles 2015, p. 10). This is particularly important as those at the top seem to be the worst offenders. To this end, the appointment of an independent ombudsman would be beneficial. The journey through the lengthy processes of the system and sometimes associated adverse experiences for IMGs could be assisted and simplified with a one-stop approach. According to recommendation 43 made by the 2012 Parliamentary Inquiry (p. xxxii): "A one-stop-shop could take on an individualised case management service for IMGs". This service should be provided by case managers who are familiar with the plethora of requirements and processes involved in the accreditation, registration and employment of IMGs. Expert staff would be empowered to work across all associated bodies and organisations involved (including the Department of Immigration and Border Protection for visa arrangements). IMGs would have a 'go to' person with whom they could become familiar and who would be focussed on negotiations and monitoring in the best interests of the IMG concerned. Case managers who experienced unfair dealings or exaggerated difficulties/delays with any part of the system would be empowered to approach the independent ombudsman on an IMG's behalf. This approach has the potential to expedite the process journey for IMGs and facilitate their employment. These initiatives represent a starting point only, but it is a good start. Hospitals, medical schools and universities must clamp down on unacceptable behaviours by enacting duty of care and the adoption of a zero-tolerance approach. Medical educators and those providing supervision must be properly trained in the effective and responsible teaching of adults. If complaints can be handled fairly by an independent/impartial ombudsman, over time, poor behaviour instances should decrease.

In the longer term, an extensive restructure of the system would be timely and contribute to culture change. Tweaking things around the edges or perhaps adding a new extra process in an effort to correct inefficiencies or problems does not constitute the real change required to tackle medicine's toxic culture. Nor does it prepare medicine to engage with disintermediation and the transformational technological revolution underway. In an environment dominated by digital, disintermediation is not just a matter of downsizing or eliminating levels within the organisation or dispensing with links in a supply chain. It also refers to: "The changing and often diminished role of traditional intermediaries…and therefore the changing relationship between individuals and institutions" (Cargnello and Flumain 2017, p. 608). The future of the Australian health system if Susskind and Susskind (2015) are correct will involve ever increasingly capable technological systems which will result in the incremental replacement of health professionals. If a member of the general public has a smart phone and a basic level of digital literacy, a growing number of medical-related services, will be readily available. This major technological shift is a global one and writing from Canada, Alami et al. (2017, p. 608) offer a warning:

> Abandon current practices and models of service, often marked by disciplinary, corporate and organisational silos as well as laws and regulations that are no longer in tune with the reality. Health systems should, because of their social responsibility, be actors (and not spectators) of the ongoing digital revolution. If this technological shift is missed, the emergence of parallel health systems, borne by new actors, is inevitable.

It is vital then that medicine in Australia keep up with, if not become a leader in, the technological revolution of medical services. Organisations are now endeavouring to work smarter and flatter. Therefore, given the impetus to address a toxic culture, in the process, this should involve major organisational restructuring to not only facilitate cultural change but also preparedness for technological advances. Following the lead taken by The Royal Australasian College of Surgeons, other colleges would do well to benchmark their plans for action with this body's initiatives. A major restructure could consider the amalgamation of the AMC and MBA which would bring about the emergence of one more streamlined body, to deal with processes such as accreditation, registration, examination and training for IMGs. To create a best practice model for efficient amalgamation would involve expert consultants and a review of other models around the world. Another beneficial move towards change is the membership of boards; in order to interrupt entrenched ideas, introduce new ways of doing things and achieve more transparency, board membership should expand. Boards should include women, IMGs, students, members of the public, educators, business leaders and technological experts. More inclusive and representative boards will provide the opportunity to progress with the input and involvement of all stakeholders. Hopefully medicine will be empowered via these suggested measures, to undertake the long road of change management. More inclusive and transparent processes invite new ways to break down old ways. Australia deserves a healthy medical culture and healthy medical professionals.

Medicine is a demanding, stressful profession which carries enormous pressures and responsibilities. Doctors often have the responsibility of life and death decisions in their hands. Many doctors are hard-working, decent human beings but clearly some are not. Patients are entitled to expect safe, uncompromised health care. Bullying behaviours cannot be tolerated as a rite of passage into medicine. Sexual harassment must be met with zero tolerance. IMGs are entitled to expect a fair and timely assessment free from discrimination and unacceptable behaviours. Many careers, hopes and aspirations have been destroyed at the hands of Australia's toxic medical culture. One doctor's, trainee's or medical student's suicide is one too many. From the anti-oppressive theoretical perspective and social justice imperative of this book: Please, no more lives torn apart.

# References

Alami, H., Gagon, M. P., & Fortin, J. P. (2017). Digital health and the challenge of health systems transformation. *Perspective*, 1–5, viewed March 26, 2018. http://dx.doi.org/10.21037/mhealth20 17.07.02.

Armstrong, P., & Britton, B. (2016). 'Nigel Farage: Arch-eurosceptic and brexit' puppet master. *CNN*, viewed November 15, 2016. http://edition.cnn.com/2016/06/24/europe/eu-referendum-ni gel-farage/index.html.

Australian Broadcasting Commission. (2016). *Much admired surgeon: Charlie Teo*. Anh's Brush with Fame, September 7, 2016. https://simkl.com/tv/609866/anhs-brush-with-fame/season-1/ep isode3.

Australian Government Department of Immigration and Border Protection. (2016). Australian Government, viewed October 5, 2016. https://www.border.gov.au.

Australian Medical Association (2016). Viewed August 25, 2016, http://www.amc.org.au/.

Baudrillard, J. (2010). *Carnival and cannibal*. Calcutta: Seagull Press.

Bacchi, C. (2009). *Analysing policy: What's the problem represented to be?*. Frenchs Forest, NSW: Pearson Australia.

Beyond Blue. (2013). *National mental health survey of doctors and medical students*, viewed October 12, 2015. www.beyondblue.org.au.

Blackshaw, T. (2010). *Key concepts in Community Studies*, Sage Key concepts series. London: Sage Publications.

Brannan, S., Campbell, R., Davies, M., English, V., Mussell, R., & Sheather, J. C. (2016). The Mediteranian refugee crisis: ethics, international law and migrant health. *Journal of Medical Ethics, 42*(4), 269–270.

Breen, S. (2008). Defending the National Honour: The history crusaders and Australia's past. In A. Gunstone (Ed.), *History, politics and knowledge: Essays in Australian Indigenous studies* (pp. 168–190). North Melbourne: Australian Scholarly Publishing Pty Ltd.

Brown, L., & Strega, S. (2005). *Research as resistance: Critical, indigenous and anti-oppressive approaches*. Toronto: Canadian Scholars' Press.

Brown, L., & Strega, S. (2015). *Research as resistance: Revisiting critical, indigenous, and anti-oppressive approaches*. Toronto: Canadian Scholars' Press.

Burton, F., & Carlen, P. (1979). *Official discourse: On discourse analysis, government publications, ideology and the state*. London: Routledge & Kegan Paul.

Campus Review. (2015). *Students want change of medical culture*. Campus Review, viewed January 12, 2016. https://www.campusreview.com.au.

Cannane, S. (2015). *A special Late line report on a French doctor who left Australia after he was the subject of repeated anonymous complaints and medical audits—was he deserving of scrutiny or was his treatment professional harassment?* Australian Broadcasting Commission, September 3, 2015, http://iview.abc.net.au/programs/latelin.

Cargnello, D. P., & Flumain, K. (2017). Canadian governance in transition: Multilevel governance in the digital era. *Canadian Public Administration, 60*(4), 605–626, viewed March 18, 2018. https://onlinelibrary.wiley.com/doi/edf/10.1111/capa.12230.

Chang, C. (2016). Who is UKIP leader Nigel Farage?. *news.com.au*, viewed November 15, 2016. http://www.news.com.au/world/europe/who-is-ukip-leader-nigel-farage/news-story/3e5f1 ccef6c2b03b91aadc8eb6c6d9eb.

Coburn, D. (2006). Medical dominance then and now: Critical reflections. *Health Sociology Review, 15*(5), 432–443.

Coburn, D., & Willis, E. (2000). The medical profession: knowledge, power, and autonomy. In G. L. Albrecht, R. Fitzpatrick, & S. C. Scrimshaw (Eds.), *Handbook of social studies in health and medicine* (pp. 377–393). London: Sage.

Darder, A., & Miron, L. F. (2006). Critical Pedagogy in a Time of Uncertainty: A call to action. In Denzin, N.K. & Girdina, M.D. *Contesting Empire/Globalising Dissent: Cultural Studies After 9/11*. Boulder, CO: Paradigm.

Denzin, N. K., & Lincoln, Y. S. (2008). Critical methodologies and Indigenous inquiry. In N. K. Denzin, Y. S. Lincoln, & L. T. Smith (Eds.), *Critical indigenous metholdologies* (pp. 1–20). Sage.

Douglas, S. (2008). The registration and accreditation of international medical graduates in Australia: A broken system or a work in progress. *People and Place, 16*(2), 28–40.

Dreyfus, M. (2017). Press conference March 21, 2017. Canberra: Parliament House. Viewed March 23, 2017, https://markdreyfus.nationbuilder.com/parliament_house_press_conference210317.

Duckett, S. (2008). The Australian health care systems: Reform, repair or replace? *Australian Health Review, 32*(2), 322–329.

Dwyer, J. (2007). *What's wrong with the global migration of health care professionals? Individual rights and international justice.* Hastings Center Report.

Eckermann, A. K., Dowd, T., Chong, E., Nixon, L., Gray, R., & Johnson, S. (2006). *Binan Goonj: Bridging cultures in Aboriginal health* (2nd ed.). Marrickville: Churchill Livingstone Elsevier.

Foley, D. (2008). An Indigenous standpoint theory. In A. Gunstone (Ed.), *History, politics and knowledge* (pp. 113–133). North Melbourne, VIC: Australian Scholarly Publishing Pty Ltd.

Foucault, M. (1985). *The use of pleasure: Vol. 2 of the history of sexuality.* New York: Pantheon Books.

Foucault, M. (1997). Subjectivity and truth. in S. Lotringer (Ed.), *The politics and truth* (pp. 147–168). Boston, MA: MIT Press.

Freidson, E. (1994). *Professionalism reborn: Theory, prophecy, and policy.* Chicago: University of Chicago Press.

Freidson, E. (2001). *Professionalism, the third logic: On the practice of knowledge.* Chicago: University of Chicago Press.

Galtung, J. (1990). Cultural violence. *Journal of Peace research, 27*, 291–305, viewed May 16, 2012. http://jpr.sagepub.com/.

Germov, (Ed.). (2014). *Second opinion* (5th ed.). South Melbourne: Oxford University Press.

Grigg, K., & Manderson, L. (2016). The Australian racism, acceptance, and cultural—Ethnocentrism scale (RACES): Item response theory findings. *International Journal for Equity in Health, 15*(49), 1–16, viewed March 9, 2017. https://doi.org/10.1186/s12939-016-0338-4, http://equityh ealthj.biomedcentral.com/articles/10.1186/s..

Gunstone, A. (2007). *Unfinished Business: The Australian formal reconciliation process.* Melbourne VIC: Australian Scholarly Publishing Pty Ltd.

Gunstone. (2017). Reconciliation, peacebuilding and Indigenous people in Australia. in H. Devere, K. Te Maiharoa & J. P. Synott (Eds.), *Peacebuilding and the rights of indigenous people: Experiences and strategies for the 21st century* (pp. 17–28). Springer International Publishing.

Haikerwal, M. (2005). *Observations from an overseas trained doctor.* Australian Medical Association, viewed April 5, 2007. http://www.ama.com.au/web.nsf/doc/WEEN-6EG7CN.

Harris, A. (2009). Overseas doctors in Australian hospitals: An ethnographic study of how degrees of difference are negotiated in medical practice. Ph.D. thesis, University of Melbourne.

Harris, A., & Guillemin, M. (2015). Notes on the medical underground: migrant doctors at the margins. *Health Sociology Review, 24*(2), 163–174, viewed March 21, 2016. http://dx.doi.org/1 0.1080/14461242.2014.999403.

Hawthorne, L., Birrell, B., & Young, D. (2004). The retention of overseas trained doctors in general practice in regional Victoria, pp. 1–100.

Hern, A. (2016). Stephen Hawking: AI will be 'either best or worst thing' for humanity. *The Guardian,* October 20, 2016.

Hill Collins, P. (2000). *Black feminist thought: Knowledge consciousness, and the politics of empowerment,* 2nd edn. New York: Routledge.

Hill Collins, P. (2010). The new politics of community. *American Sociological Review, 75*(1), 7–30, viewed September 6, 2012. https://doi.org/10.1177/0003122410363293, via Sage (dowloaded from asr.sagepub.com at Adelaide theological library). http://asr.sagepub.com.

Hill Collins, P., & Bilge, S. (2016). *Intersectionality.* Cambridge, UK: Polity Press.

Hill Collins, P., & Solomos, J. (Eds.). (2010). *The sage handbook of race and ethnic studies.* Los Angeles: Sage Publications.

Hirst, J. (2014). *Australian history in 7 questions*. Collingwood Vic: Black Inc.

Hook, D. (2001). Discourse, knowledge, materiality, history: Foucault and discourse analysis. *Theory and Psychology, 11*(4), 521–547.

Iredale, (2009). Luring overseas trained doctors to Australia: Issues of training, regulating and trading. *International Migration, 47*(4), 31–64.

Kahn, F. A., Chikkatagaiah, S., & Shafiullah, M. (2015). IMGs in the UK: A systematic review of their acculturation and adaptation. *Journal of International Migration and Integration, 16*(3), 743–759, viewed October 13, 2016. http://link.springer.com/article/10.1.

Keleher, H. (2016). The medical profession in Australia. In E. Willis, L. Reynolds, & H. Keleher (Eds.), *Understanding the Australian health care system,* (3rd ed., pp. 395–408). Chatswood, NSW: Elsevier.

Kidd, R. (2008). Wealth and poverty. In A. Gunstone (Ed.), *History, politics and knowledge: Essays in Australian Indigenous studies* (pp. 148–167). North Melbourne, VIC: Australian Scholarly Publication Pty Ltd.

Knowles, R. (2015). *Expert advisory group draft report on discrimination, bullying and sexual harassment*. Royal Australasian College of Surgeons. Viewed 15 October 2015. https://www.surgeons.org/media/2204568/eag-report-to-racs-draft-08-sept-2015.pdf.

Kunz, E. F. (1975). *The intruders: Refugee doctors in Australia*. Canberra: Australian National University Press.

Lueck, K., Due, C., & Augoustinos, M. (2015). Neoliberalism and nationalism: Representations of asylum seekers in the Australian mainstream news media. *Discourse and Society, 26*(5), 608–629, viewed April 25, 2017. https://doi.org/10.1177/0957926515581159, https://www.das.sagepub.com.

Macias, T. (2015). On the footsteps of Foucault: Doing Foucauldian discourse analysis in social justice research. In S. Strega & L. Brown (Eds.), *Research as resistance: Revisiting critical, Indigenous, and anti-oppressive approaches* (2nd ed., pp. 221–242). Toronto: Canadian Scholars' Press.

Maley, W. (2016). Australia's refugee policy: Domestic politics and diplomatic consequences. *Australian Journal of International Affairs, 70*(6), 670–680, viewed November 8, 2016, via Routledge Taylor and Francis group (Flinders University). http://www.tandfonline.com.exproxy.

McDermott, Q. (2015). *At their Mercy*. Four Corners, Australian Broadcasting Commission. viewed May 5, 2015, www.abc.net.au/4corners/at-their-mercy/6488010..

Medical Deans Australia and New Zealand. (2017). *Inherent requirements for studying medicine in Australia and New Zealand*. viewed September 10, 2017, https://medcaldeansorg.au/md/2018/07/Inherent-Requirements-FINAL-statement_July 2017. pdf.

Mills, C. W. (1959). *The sociological imagination*. Oxford: Oxford University Press.

Moreton-Robinson, A. (2004). Whiteness, epistemology and Indigenous representation. In A. Moreton-Robinson (Ed.), *Whitening race: Essays in social and cultural criticism* (pp. 75–88). Canberra: Aboriginal Studies Press for the AIATSIS.

Murray, R. (2017). Letter to the editor: Medical deans are committed to student health and wellbeing. *Medical Observer*, viewed March 26, 2018. http://www.medicaldeans.org.au/wp-content/uploads/Medical-Observer_Letter-to-the-Editor_RMurray_22-Nov-2017.pdf.

Newman, J., & Head, B. (2017). The national context of wicked problems: Comparing policies on gun violence in the US, Canada, and Australia. *Journal of Comparative Policy Analysis: Research and Practice, 19*(1), 40–53.

OECD. (2015). *Chapter 3: Changing patterns in the international migration of doctors and nurses to OECD countries* . In International Migration Outlook. Immigrant health workers in OECD countries in the broader context of highly skilled migration. https://www.oecd.org/migration/mig/41515701pdf..

One Nation Party. (2016). Viewed November 11, 2016. http://www.onenation.com.au.

Plage, S., Willing, I., Skrbis, Z., Woodward, I. (2016). Australiannes as fairness: Implications for cosmopolitan encounters. *Journal of Sociology, 1*(6), 1–16, viewed February 9, 2017, via Sage (Flinders University, South Australia). http://jos.sagepub.com.

Potts, K., & Brown, L. (2015). Becoming an anti-oppressive researcher. In S. Strega & L. Brown (Eds.), *Research as resistance: revisiting critical, Indigenous, and anti-oppressive approaces* (2nd ed., pp. 17–41). Toronto: Canadian Scholars' Press.

Reid, J. S., Taylor, K., & Hayes, C. (2016). Indigenous health systems and services. In L. Reynolds, H. Keleher, & E. Willis (Eds.), *Understanding the Australian Health Care System* (pp. 153–166). Chatswood: Elsevier.

Riley, A. (2016. Same old rhetoric cannot justify banning refugees from Australia. *The Conversation*, viewed November 17, 2016. http://www.theconversation.com/same-old-rhetoric-cannot-justify-banning-refugees-from-australia-67923.

Sefa Dei, G. J. (2008). Race, difference, and the discourse of intersectionality. in *Racists beware: Uncovering racial politics in the post modern society* (pp. 81–91). The Netherlands: Sense Publishers.

Sen, A. (2010). *The idea of justice*. United Kingdom: Penguin.

Sen, A. (2016). Reason and justice: The optimal and the maximal. *The Royal Institute of Philosophy, 92*(1), 5–19, viewed July 23, 2017. https://doi.org/10.1017/s0031819116000309.

Sherden, A., & Cannane, S. (2015). *Neurosurgeon Dr Charlie Teo says 'bullying culture' in medicine destroying lives, backs call for inquiry*. September 4, 2015 edn, ABC News, October 24, 2016. http://www.abc.net.au/news/2015-09-04-abcnews(Australian-dr-charlie-teo-backs-call-for-medical-complaints-inquiry/6751402.

Smith, S. D. (2008). The global workforce shortages and the migration of medical professions: The Australian response. *Australia and New Zealand Health Policy, 5*(7), viewed June 6, 2009. http://www.anzhealthpolicy.com/content/5/1/7.

Standing, G. (2011). *The Precariat: The new dangerous class*. London: Bloomsbury Academic.

Strega, S. (2015). The view from the poststructural margins: Epistemology and methodology reconsidered. In S. Strega & L. Brown (Eds.), *Research as resistance, revisiting critical, Indigenous, and anti-oppressive approaches* (2nd ed., pp. 119–152). Toronto: Canadian Scholars' Press.

Sullivan, M. (2016). *The patient as agent of health and health care: Autonomy in patient-centered care of chronic conditions*. United Kingdom: Oxford University Press.

Susskind, R., & Susskind, D. (2015). *The future of the professions: How technology will transform the work of human experts*. New York: Oxford University Press.

The Senate Community Affairs References Committee. (2016). *Medical complaints process in Australia*, Canberra, Viewed January 5, 2017. https://www.aph.gov.au/Parliamentary_Business/Committees/Senate/Community_Affairs/MedicalComplaints45.

Toader, E., & Sfetcu, L. (2013). The medical migration: Experiences and perspectives of medical students for the professional career. *Revista de cercetare si interventie sociala, 40*, 124–136.

Twohig, J. (2016). The complementary and alternative health care system in Australia. In E. Willis, L. Reynolds, & H. Keleher (Eds.), *Understanding the Australian health care system* (pp. 207–224). Chatswood: Elsevier.

Wang, D. (2017). *Foucault and the smart city*. Paper presented to Design for Next: 12th EAD Conference, Sapienza University of Rome, April 12–24, 2017. http://eprints.lancs.ac.uk?85521/1/DfN-full-paper-DW.

Ward, S., & Outram, S. (2016). Medicine: In need of culture change. *International Medical Journal, 46*(1), 112–116, viewed April 3, 2017. http://onlinelibrary.wiley.com/doi/10.1111/imj.12954.

Willis, E. (1989). *Medical dominance: The division of labour in Australian health care*, revised edn. North Sydney: Allen & Unwin.

Willis, E. (2006). Introduction: Taking stock of medical dominance. *Health Sociology Review, 15*(5), 421–431.

Willis, E., Reynolds, L., & Keleher, H. (Eds.). (2016). *Understanding the Australian health care system* (3rd ed.). Chatswood NSW: Elsevier.

# Appendix A

**House of Representatives Standing Committee on Health and Ageing 2012,** *Inquiry into Registration Processes and Support for Overseas Trained Doctors*, **the Parliament of the Commonwealth of Australia, Canberra**

|  | Submission |
|---|---|
| Dr A | 66 |
| Dr Anon | 15 |
| Australian Medical Council | 42 |
| Dr BJ | 26 |
| Dr Da | 6 |
| Dr D | 111 |
| Dr G | 31 |
| Dr Go | 25 |
| Dr I | 134 |
| Dr L | 118 |
| National Rural Health Alliance | 113 |
| Dr N | 153 |
| Dr S | 150 |
| Dr St: *Official Committee Hansard*: public hearing 10 March 2011 | |
| Dr T | 102 |
| Dr W | 68 |

© Springer Nature Singapore Pte Ltd. 2019
V. A. Pascoe, *Australia's Toxic Medical Culture*,
https://doi.org/10.1007/978-981-13-2426-0

## The Senate Community Affairs References Committee 2016, *Medical Complaints Process in Australia*, Canberra

<table>
<tr><td></td><td>Submission</td></tr>
<tr><td>Australian Indigenous Doctors' Association</td><td>8</td></tr>
<tr><td>Australian Medical Association</td><td>9</td></tr>
<tr><td>Australian Medical Students' Association</td><td>10</td></tr>
<tr><td>Ms B: Official Committee Hansard:<br>   public hearing 1 November 2016</td><td></td></tr>
<tr><td>Dr F: Official Committee Hansard:<br>   public hearing 1 November 2016</td><td></td></tr>
<tr><td>Health Care Consumers' Association</td><td>16</td></tr>
<tr><td>Dr K: Health Practitioners Australia Reform Association:<br>Official Committee Hansard: public hearing 1 November 2016</td><td></td></tr>
<tr><td>Prof. S: Official Committee Hansard:<br>   public hearing 1 November 2016</td><td></td></tr>
</table>

# Bibliography

Anderson, S. (2016). *Who will come to Australia*, viewed October 19, 2016, http://www.abc.net.au/news/2016-03-17/immigration-minister-peter-dutton/7254828.

Australian Bureau of Statistics. (2013). *Australian Demographic Statistics: March 2013*, Australian Bureau of Statistics, viewed November 12, 2016, http://www.abs.gov.au/AUSSTATS/abs@nsf/Lookup/3101.0.

Australian Competition and Consumer Commission and the Australian Health Workforce Officials' Committee. (2005). *Review of Australian specialist medical colleges*. Commonwealth of Australia, Canberra.

Australian Doctors Trained Overseas Association (ADTOA). (2012). *Passionate cries from parliament: There needs to be a fairer go for overseas trained doctors*, viewed May 25, 2011, http://www.adtoa.org.au.

Australian Health Practitioner Regulation Agency. (2014). *AHPRA responds to Parliamentary Committee Report*, 1, AHPRA, Sydney, March 12, 2014, https://www.aphra.gov.au/News.

Australian Medical Association. (2011). *Submission 42: Registration and support for overseas trained doctors*, by Australian Medical Council.

Australian Medical Association. (2007). *Tackling wicked problems: A public policy perspective*, by Australian Public Service Commission, Commonwealth of Australia.

Bauman, Z. (2013). In Z. Bauman (Ed.), *Community: Seeking safety in an Insecure World*. Berlin: Wiley, viewed April 10, 2017 (ProQuest Ebook Central), http://ebookcentral.proquest.com.ezproxy.flinders.edu.au/lib/flinders/detail.action?docID=1187719.

Brannan, S., Campbell, R., Davies, M., English, V., Mussell, R. l., & Sheather, J. C. (2016). The Mediteranian refugee crisis: Ethics, international law and migrant health. *Journal of Medical Ethics, 42*(4), 269–270.

Campbell, D., Siddique, H., Kirk, A., & Meikle, J. (2015). NHS hires up to 3,000 foreign-trained doctors in a year to plug staff shortages. *The Guardian*, January 29, 2015.

Castles, S., Foster, W., Iredale, R., & Withers, G. (1998). *Immigration and Australia: Myths and realities*. St Leonards: Allen & Unwin in Conjunction with the Housing Industry Association Ltd.

Crenshaw, K. (1989). Demarginalizing the intersection of race and sex: A black feminist critique of antidiscrimination doctrine, feminist theory, and antiracist politics. *University of Chicago Legal Forum, 14,* 538–554.

Demianyk, G. (2016). Nigel Farage dismisses Anti-Donald Trump and Brexit protestors as 'professionals' too lazy to vote. *The Huffington post*, viewed November 14, 2016, http://www.huffingtonpost.co.uk/entry/nigel-farage-donald-trump-protests_uk_5828921de4b09ac74c528c04.

Denzin, N. K. (2007). The Sage handbook of grounded theory. In A. Bryant & K. Charmaz (Eds.).

Department of Immigration and Border Protection. (2016). *Australian government*, Canberra, October 20, 2016, https://www.pm.gov.au/media/2016-10-30/joint-pressconference-minister-immigrationand-border-protection.

Donini, A., Monsutti, A., & Scalettaris, G. (2016). *Afghans on the move: Seeking protection and refuge in Europe. In this journey I died several times; in Afghanistan you only die once*, Geneva.

Donnelly, L. (2014). UK has fewer doctors than almost every EU country. *Telegraph*, December 2014, Health.

Foucault, M. (1972). *The archaeology of knowledge*. London: Tavistock.

Freidson, E. (1994). *Professionalism reborn: Theory, prophecy, and policy*. Chicago: University of Chicago Press.

Fry, R. G. (1982). *The recognition of overseas qualifications in Australia*, Canberra.

Hall, S. (1979). The great moving right show. *Marxism Today*.

Hawthorne, L. (2013). International medical migration: What is the future for Australia? *Medical Journal of Australia*, 18–21, viewed May 2, 2018, https://doi.org/10.5694/mjao12.10088, https://www.mja.com.au/system/files/issues/001_03_230712/haw10088C_fm.pdf.

Hill Collins, P. (2013). *On intellectual activism*. Philadelphia: Temple University Press.

Hocking, D. (2010). Sorry seemed to be the hardest word. In A. Gunstone (Ed.), *Over a decade of despair: The Howard government and indigenous affairs* (pp. 51–74). North Melbourne: Australian Scholarly Publishing Pty. Ltd.

Hoekje, B. J. (2007). Medical discourse and ESP courses for IMGs. *English for specific purposes, 26*(3), 327–343.

Human Rights and Equal Opportunities Commission. (1997). *Bringing them home: Report of the National Inquiry into the separation of Aboriginal and Torres Strait Islander Children from their Families*, Sydney.

Human Rights and Equal Opportunity Commission. (1991). *The experiences of overseas medical practitioners in Australia: An analysis in the light of the Racial Discrimination Act 1975*, Sydney.

Innes, J. E., & Booher, D. E. (2016). Collaborative Relationality as a strategy for working with Wicked Problems. *Landscape and Urban Planning, 154*, 1–132, viewed May 1, 2017, https://doi.org/10.1016/j.landurplan.2016.03.016, via Sciencedirect.com, http://www.sciencedirect.com/science/journal/01692046/154/sup/C.

Keller, R. (2017). Has critique run out of steam?—On discourse research a critical inquiry. *Qualitative Inquiry, 23*(1), 58–68, viewed May 6, 2017, https://doi.org/10.1177/1077800416657103, http://journals.sagepub.com.exproxy.flinders.edu.au.

Kidd, M., & Braun, F. (1992). *Problems encountered by overseas-trained doctors migrating to Australia*. Canberra: Bureau of Immigration Research.

Kovach, M. (2005). Emerging from the margins: Indigenous methodologies. In L. Brown & S. Strega (Eds.), *Research as resistance: Critical, indigenous, and anti-oppressive approaches* (pp. 19–36), Toronto: Canadian Scholars' Press.

Lavery, J. V. (2016). 'Wicked problems', community engagement and the need for an implementation science for research ethics. *Journal of Medical Ethics, 0*(0), 1–2, viewed April 21, 2017, https://doi.org/10.1136/medethics-2016-103573, http://jme.bmj.com.

Law Council of Australia. (2008). *Clarke inquiry into the case of Dr Mohamed Haneef*, Canberra.

Legislative Council Legal and Social Issues Legislation Committee. (2014). *Inquiry into the Performance of the Australian Health Practitioner Regulation Agency*, Parliament of Victoria, Victoria.

Li, S. S. Y., Liddell, B. J., & Nickerson, A. (2016). The relationship between post-migration stress and psychological disorders in refugees and asylum seekers. *Current Psychiatry Reports, 18* (82), 1–9, viewed April 19, 2017, http://cugmhp.org/wp-content/uploads/2017/03/The-Relationship-Between-Post-Migration-Stress-And-Psychological-Disorders-In-Refugees-And-Assylum-Seekers.

Losoncz, I. (2017). Transforming lives and institutions: The structural inclusion and institutional engagement of refugee migrants in Australia. *REGNET Research Paper*, p. 28, viewed May 9, 2017, https://doi.org/10.2139/ssrn.2929559, https://ssrn.com/abstract=2929559.

Malekpour, M., Fatehizadeh, M., Hashemian, S., & Velayati, A. (2009). Retaining health manpower in developing countries. *The Lancet, 374*(9686), 291–292, viewed November 2, 2012, http://www.thelancet.com/.

Malin, M. (1997). An anti-racism teacher education program. In S. Harris & M. Malin (Eds.), *Indigenous education: Historical, moral and practical tales*. Darwin: Northern Territory University Press.

McIlroy, T. (2016). Immigration minister Peter Dutton says new refugee ban will stop country hopping. *The Age*, viewed November 21, 2016, http://www.theage.cpm.au/federal-politics-news/immigration-minister-peter-dutton-says-new-refugee-ban-will-stop-country-hopping-20161030-gse8jx.html.

McQuillan, J. C. (2016). Beyond the analytic of finitude: Kant, Heidegger, Foucault. *Foucault Studies, 21*, 184–199, viewed May 5, 2017, https://rauli.cbs.dk/index.php/foucault-studies/index.

Metzger, J., Soneryd, L., & Tamm-Hallstrom, K. (2017). 'Power' is that which remains to be explained: Dispelling the Ominous dark matter of Capital Planning Studies. *Planning Theory, 16*(2), 203–222, viewed May 9, 2017, https://doi.org/10.1177/1473095215622502, http://www.journals.sagepub.com/home/plt.

Miernowski, J. (2016). In J. Miernowski (Ed.), *Early modern Humanism and postmodern Antihumanism in dialogue*. Basingstoke: Palgrave Macmillan, viewed May 5, 2017, https://doi.org/10.1007/978-3-318-32276-6.

Mills, C. W. (1956). *The power elite*. New York: Oxford University Press.

Moran, A. (2016). *The Public Life of Australia: Multiculturalism, Building a Diverse Nation*, Berlin: Springer, viewed May 9, 2017, https://doi.org/10.1007/978-3-319-45126-8-6, https://books.google.com.aubook?id=izSgDQAAQBAJ&redir-esc=y.

Nunn, C. (2017). Negotiating National (non) belongings: Vietnamese Australians in ethno/multicultural Australia. *Identities, Global Studies in Culture and Power, 24*(2), 216–235, viewed May 6, 2017, https://doi.org/10.1080/1070289x.2015.1096273, http://www.tandfonline.com.

O'Leary, T. (2016). New books "by" Foucault review: Speech begins after death. *Foucault Studies, 21*, 231–237, viewed May 7, 2017, https://rauli.cbs.dk/index.php/foucault-studies/index.

Paradies, Y., Ben, J., Denson, N., Elias, A., Priest, M., & Pieterse, A. (2015). Racism as a determinant of health: A systemic review and meta-analysis. *PLOS ONE Journals, 10*(9), 1–48, viewed March 14, 2017, http://journals.plos.org/plosone/article?id=10.1371/journal.pone.0138511.

Phillips, J., Klapdor, M., & Simon-Davies, J. (2010). Migration to Australia since federation: A guide to the statistics, pp. 1–29, viewed May 23, 2017, http://www.aph.gov.au/About_Parliament/Parliament_Departments/Parliamentary_Library/pubs/BN/1011/MigrationPopulation.

Pourmokhtari, N. (2017). Protestation and mobilization in the Middle East and North Africa: A Foucauldian model. *Foucault Studies, 22*, 177–207, viewed May 6, 2017, https://doi.org/10.22439/fs.v0i0.5240.

Productivity Commission. (2005). *Australia's Health Workforce: Research Report*, Australian Government, Canberra.

Rawlings, V. (2017). *Gender regulation, Violence and Social Hierarchies in School: 'Sluts', 'Gays' and 'Scrubs'*, Palgrave Macmillan, UK, viewed May 7, 2017 (Flinders University South Australia), Downloaded Springer.com.exproxy.flinders.edu.au/static/pdf.

Redhead, S. (2015). *Football and accelerated culture: This modern sporting life*. London: Routledge Research in Sport, Culture and Society, Routledge Taylor & Francis Group.

Roffee, J. A. (2016). Rhetoric, Aboriginal Australians and the Northern Territory intervention: A socio-legal investigation into pre-legislative argumentation. *International Journal for Crime, Justice and Social Democracy*, viewed April 22, 2017, http://www.healthinfonet.ecu.edu.au/uploads/resources/3113-31113.pdf.

Roose, J., & Dietz, H. (2016). *Social theory and social movements: Mutual inspirations.* In J. Roose & H. Dietz (Eds.), Berlin: Springer, viewed May 5, 2017, https://doi.org/10.1007/978-3-658-13381-8.

Schech, S., & Haggis, J. (2000). *Culture and development.* Oxford: Blackwell publishers.

Schotel, B. (2012). *On the right of exclusion: Law, ethics and immigration policy.* New York: Routledge.

Senate Finance and Public Administration References Committee. (2011). *The Administration of Health Practitioner Registration by the Australian Health Practitioner Regulation Agency (AHPRA)*, Parliament of Australia, Canberra.

Shute, T. (2017). Monochrome racism: Aboriginal and Non-Aboriginal attitudes towards racism in the 21st century. *Ethos, 25*(1), 7–15, viewed May 9, 2017, http://search.informit.com.au.exproxy.flinders.edu.au/documentsummary:dn=780626774622224;res=IELHSS.

Sidhu, R. (2017). Navigating unfreedoms and re-imagining ethical counter-conducts: Caring about Refugees and Asylum Seekers. *Educational Philosophy and Theory, 49*(3), 1–12, viewed May 6, 2017, https://doi.org/10.1080/00131857.2016.1225558, http://www.tandfonline.com.

Stanner, W. E. H. (1969). *After the dreaming. Black and White Australians: An Anthropologist's view*, Sydney.

The National Population Council. (1988). *Recognition of Overseas Qualifications and Skills: Report by a working party*, Department of Immigration, Local government and ethnic affairs, Canberra.

The New South Wales Committee of Inquiry. (1989). *Recognition of Overseas Qualifications*, Sydney.

The World Bank. (2011). *Physicians per 1,000*, May 17, 2016, http://www.data.worldbank.org/indicator/SH.MED.PHYS.ZS.

United Nations. (1948). Universal Declaration of Human Rights, viewed November 30, 2012, http://www.un.org/en/documents/udhr/.

Vandaele, E. (2016). What is an author, indeed: Michel Foucault in translation. *Perspectives: Studies in Translatology, 24*(1), 76–92, viewed May 5, 2017, https://doi.org/10.1080/0907676x.2015.1047386.

Waddell, S. (2016). Societal change systems: A framework to address wicked problems. *Journal of Applied Behavioural Science, 52*(4), 422–449, viewed October 25, 2016 (Downloaded from Flinders University), http://jab.sagepub.com.

Waddock, S. (2013). The wicked problems of global sustainability need wicked (good) leaders and wicked (good) collaborative solutions. *Journal of Management for Global Sustainability, 1*, 91–111, viewed May 1, 2017, http://journals.ateneo.edu/ojs/jmgs/article/viewFile/JM2013.01106/1637.

Walsh, A., Banner, S., Schabort, I., Armson, H., Bowmer, I., & Granata, B. (2011). *International medical graduates—Current issues*, Canada.

World Health Organisation. (2011). *The WHO code of global practice on the international recruitment of health personnel*, WHO, viewed October 20, 2016, http://www.who.int/hrh/migraion/code/practice/en/.

World Health Organisation. (2016a). 'Medical and nursing students' intentions to work abroad or in rural areas: a cross-sectional survey in Asia and Africa. *Bulletin of the WHO*, viewed October 12, 2016, http://www.who.int/bulletin.

World Health Organisation. (2016b). *Royal College of Surgeons Ireland Workforce alliance*, 30 June 2016 Ed., World Health Organisation (WHO), October 12, 2016, http://www.who.int/workforcealliance/brain-drain=gain/irish_doctor-emigration-chalenge/en/.

Xenophon, N. (2016). *Senate inquiry into medical complaints regime: health complaints system under the microscope*, Canberra, February 2, 2016, http://www.nickxenophon.com.au/media/releases/show/senate-inquiry-into-medical-complaints-regime/.

Zajda, J., & Ozdowski, S. (2017). *Globalisation, comparative education and policy research.* J. Zajda & S. Ozdowski (Eds.), Berlin: Springer, viewed May 9, 2017, https://doi.org/10.1007/978-94-024-0871-3.

Zamora, D., & Behrent, M. C. (2016). *Foucault and Neoliberalism*. New York: Wiley.

Zmerli, S., & Van Der Meer, T. W. G. (2017). In S. Zmerli & T. W. G. Van Der Meer (Eds.), *Handbook on Political Trust.* Cheltenham. UK: Edward Elgar Publishing, viewed May 9, 2017, https://doi.org/10.4337/9781782545118, https://books.google.com/books?isbn=1782545115.